The Pre-PA Guide to: Applying to Physician Assistant School with a Low GPA

Advice, Tips, & Strategies From a Former Low GPA Applicant

Samora Charles, PA-C

A GOSHEN PUBLISHERS BOOK VIRGINIA

The Pre-PA Guide to:
Applying to Physician Assistant School with a Low GPA

Advice, Tips, & Strategies
From a Former Low GPA Applicant

ISBN: 978-1-7370949-0-6

Library of Congress Cataloging-in-Publication Data

Published in 2022 by:

GOSHEN PUBLISHERS LLC
P.O. Box 1562, Stephens City, Virginia, USA
www.GoshenPublishers.com

Our books may be purchased in bulk for promotional, educational, or business use. For inquiries please contact the publisher via email: Agents@GoshenPublishers.com.

First Edition 2022

Cover designed by Goshen Publishers LLC

Printed in the United States of America

This book is dedicated to my husband, who has been my #1 supporter and rock throughout the years while I worked towards achieving my dream career

My circle of family and friends who saw greatness in me even when I did not see it in myself

And lastly, to all those who doubted me. Because if it were not for you, I may have never put forth the effort to prove that I am capable of accomplishing anything I set my mind to, including becoming a physician assistant.

Table of Contents

Start Here

DEAR PRE-PA

Dear Reader,

You may be questioning whether or not you should pursue the physician assistant career. Perhaps you started to look into it and have heard all about how competitive it is to get accepted to PA school. Maybe you attended an open house or checked out a few PA school requirements, and became discouraged because your GPA does not meet the listed minimum accepted. More than likely, you are someone who experienced some difficulty during undergrad, and were told by an advisor, counselor, or faculty member that your grades simply won't make the cut. It could even be that you were told to choose a different career path, even though you desire to become a PA.

I want you to know I get it. I once had those same feelings of self-doubt not so long ago. After my first round of rejections from PA schools, fourteen to be exact, I felt lost, disappointed, and defeated. I started to wonder if I would always be haunted by my past academic failures. As an applicant who was once academically dismissed from college after failing multiple classes, I'm here to tell you my PA journey has been an uphill battle. At times, I was not even sure if I would *ever* achieve my dream career. But I was determined to keep my past from affecting my future.

It took three application cycles before I was finally able to get accepted to PA school. I made many mistakes along the way and wasted hundreds of dollars in application fees because there were no resources available to steer applicants like me in the right direction. This is precisely why I decided to take the lessons I learned and create a detailed and comprehensive guide specifically for non-traditional and/or low GPA applicants like me.

It is my hope that this book will serve as a blueprint to you, no matter where you are on the journey to becoming a PA. My goal is to help clear up any misconceptions you may have, and provide you with the understanding you need to help you formulate the best plan for you. Like I tell my mentees, it will take hard work, dedication, and patience, but you can make yourself a competitive applicant by utilizing the tools in this book.

I currently work as a multispecialty Surgical PA-C at one of the top hospital systems in the country. If I could accomplish this dream, in spite of all my failures and mistakes, so can you.

Sincerely,
Samora Charles

Introduction

"We regret to inform you that you have not been selected to interview for a seat in our PA program. Each year, we receive hundreds of applications from qualified candidates..."

It was usually at this point I stopped reading, feeling the sting of tears start to form in my eyes at yet another rejection. What was I doing wrong? Why couldn't I get programs to see that I was both committed and capable of becoming a physician assistant?

As I began to research and move through one application cycle to the next, I realized it was not just one thing that was keeping me from being accepted. There were actually several areas of my application profile that needed to be refined, so I could show admission committees I was at least worthy of an interview.

When I was a pre-PA student, there were very few resources available to a low GPA, non-traditional applicant like myself. I had to learn everything the old-fashioned way: through trial and error. These days, there seems to be an abundance of YouTube channels, Instagram pages, books, and blogs that discuss different areas of the PA school application process, but most are geared towards the typical or average PA school applicant. What about everyone else?!

After I was academically dismissed from college my sophomore year, I had to work hard to get myself back into school, fix my GPA, and improve the other components of my application that PA programs assess when selecting qualified candidates. These pages address all the difficulties I faced and offer guidance from start to finish on your own journey to becoming a PA. After reading this book, you should have a clear understanding of where to begin, what your options are, and how you can make yourself a competitive, worthy applicant, no matter what anyone else tells you.

What's different about this book?

Well, for one, I was once in your shoes. I know firsthand how confusing and frustrating this process can be, which is why my goal is not to provide generic advice. Each section of this book is explained in detail and examples are provided for even more clarity. In addition to the helpful information found in each chapter, the FAQ and Appendix section also offer you even more value. I recommend you start reading from the very beginning so that you can ensure you are learning all there is to know. (What's that saying? "You don't know what you don't know.")

I also want to make clear that my intentions are not to sell you a dream or a fairy tale. The fact remains, the PA school application process has become increasingly competitive, and even those with stellar grades may have to apply more than once. However, I firmly believe that through hard work, perseverance, and most importantly patience, you can ultimately gain acceptance.

I applied to PA school three consecutive application cycles before I was accepted to not one but two PA programs, and was waitlisted at two others. As a PA student, I actively participated in my program's interviews and learned even more about the PA school admissions process from various program faculty and staff. These days, I happily serve as a pre-PA mentor and am proud to say that through my experiences, I have helped countless students gain acceptance to PA school.

While I love helping applicants of various backgrounds, I can honestly say that those who fall in the low GPA, non-traditional, or reapplicant category are the ones that I favor the most. If you identify as any or all of these, I want you to know that this book was written with you in mind. If you still have questions after reading this book, you can email me: info@samoracharles.com or message me on Instagram: @sammiesupageek.

Part 1:

The Basics

Chapter 1:
Why PA School?

Please Note: 'PA School' will be used interchangeably with 'PA Programs' throughout this book.

I am one of those who thinks there is value in understanding the origin of things, so that you can fully comprehend the challenges, prospects, and opportunities that lie ahead. As such, it only seems right that I start this book off by sharing just a little bit of history about the physician assistant (PA) profession.

The PA profession was created as a solution to the shortage of primary care providers back in the 1960s. A doctor by the name of Eugene A. Stead Jr. came up with the brilliant idea to model the "fast-track" training that was utilized during WWII to quickly train doctors and apply this method to the academic standards of PA education. He recruited four Navy Hospital Corpsmen as part of his inaugural class at Duke University in 1965. It is important to note that they each had extensive background medical experience gained through their service in the Navy. Under the tutelage of Dr. Stead, these four men successfully completed the PA program in 1967 and became the first physician assistants in the United States.

Fun Fact: The designation 'PA-C', which indicates a PA has passed the national certifying exam known as the PANCE, was not established until the year 1975.

A lot has changed for the PA profession since the 1960s. Gone are the days where PAs solely functioned under the direct supervision of a medical doctor. Although PAs are still required by law to have a supervising physician, typically this is in name only and not in actual practice. Many PAs practice team-based care and work collaboratively with doctors and other healthcare professionals to provide care to patients. However, their medical knowledge and clinical training also allows them to practice autonomously and perform a variety of tasks such as:

- Perform patient assessments and physical examinations
- Treat and diagnose patients
- Prescribe medications and other forms of treatments
- Order and interpret lab tests, imaging, and other studies
- Perform medical procedures and interventions
- Provide patient education
- Participate in medical research

Although primary care is still the primary focus of most PA programs, many PA school graduates are finding opportunities to practice medicine within a broad range of specialties (see Appendix A for a full listing). This is largely based on the fact that employers who hire PAs typically report better productivity and increased revenue, but more importantly, improved access to patient care. The profession continues to grow rapidly and has consistently ranked high on the list of best careers in healthcare and medicine overall. Don't believe me? Just ask Google!

Now that we have some of the history out of the way, let's get into the nitty gritty of PA School and the typical requirements.

Quick Facts about PA Programs

- As of October 2021, there are 277 ARC-PA accredited PA Programs in the U.S.[1]
- CASPA stands for Centralized Application Service for Physician Assistants and is the application system most PA programs will utilize to accept applications
- The majority of PA schools are full-time programs which can take anywhere from two to three years to complete
- There are also part-time, online, and (accelerated) dual degree PA program options available[2]
- PA programs are taught at the graduate level and students will receive a master's degree upon completion

---

[1] ARC-PA stands for the Accreditation Review Commission on Education for the Physician Assistant and is the accrediting agency for PA Programs that defines the standards of PA education and ensures their continued compliance. In other words, programs have to answer to them to keep their accreditation status.

[2] Dual degree options include a combined bachelor and master's degree in physician assi""stant studies (BS/MS), as well as a combined public health degree (PA/MPH).

- PA programs typically split the educational training into two parts: didactic and clinical

PA School Requirements Snapshot

Bachelor's Degree

You must have a completed bachelor's degree before you begin PA school. However, this does not mean you need to wait to apply, especially if your degree is near completion and you have fulfilled the other prerequisite requirements for the program.

PA programs do not require applicants to have a specific undergraduate major, as long as they have completed the prerequisite coursework.

Prerequisite Coursework
Although there is some variation between PA programs and their required academic coursework, almost all will have the following courses listed as an **absolute** requirement:

- General Biology I and II with lab
- General Chemistry I and II with lab
- Anatomy and Physiology I and II with lab
- Microbiology with lab
- Statistics
- Psychology

There are additional courses that are listed as either required, recommended, or suggested depending on the program, but we will get into the specifics of those in Part 2 of this book.

Healthcare Experience

Many programs will require applicants to have prior experience in healthcare. Remember how I pointed out at the beginning of this chapter that the four Navy Hospital Corpsmen had background medical experience? We probably have them to thank (or not thank) for this requirement.

The most preferable type of experience is often classified as direct PCE, otherwise known as direct patient care experience. Programs will vary on if they require a set minimum number of hours of PCE, paid vs unpaid experience, and/or preferred job type or title.

The other type of healthcare experience is classified as experience obtained in a healthcare setting, but does not involve the direct hands-on care of patients. Think medical billing, medical sales rep, or hospital volunteer for this category.

This is one of the most important requirements for PA admissions which is why I go into further detail about the specifics in Chapter 10.

Strong Academic History

And now we arrive at the very subject of this book. What exactly classifies an applicant as having a strong academic history? If you have ever asked someone what it takes to get into PA school or have already begun the research, I am sure you have heard or read that you must have earned all As and Bs throughout your undergraduate education, have well above a 3.0 GPA, and if you have ever received a C or below in any course, especially a science course, you should not even bother and pick a different career. Sound about right?

In fact, most programs have a way of driving the above points home by stating somewhere in the requirements or FAQ section of their website something along the lines of the following:

"The average undergraduate cumulative GPA of our most competitive applicants is around 3.5 or greater."

As a low GPA applicant myself, statements like the above were basically a crushing blow to my spirit. It took time for me to really comprehend what programs were looking for in this category, and the tools I learned are the foundation of what this book is based on.

But before I get too carried away, I do want to point out that there are other items PA schools may require as part of the application process such as standardized tests, essays, letters of recommendation (LORs), and PA shadowing, all of which will be covered in detail in the later chapters.

Now that you know a little bit more about the history of the PA profession, and the general admission requirements for PA school, let's move on to the more specific information you need to know to make yourself a competitive applicant, beginning with Chapter 2.

CHAPTER 2:
DEFINING NON-TRADITIONAL & LOW GPA APPLICANTS

I was both a non-traditional and low GPA applicant who was ultimately able to be accepted to PA school.

Let me begin by stating the following: the terms non-traditional applicant and low GPA applicant are not mutually exclusive. What I mean by this is although they are two separate identifiers, they can at times apply to the same applicant.

In short, non-traditional applicants are usually those who did not follow a linear path to PA school. Most often, they can be classified as any of the following:

- Second or third degree students
- Career changers
- Having gaps in education
- Older students (think +30 y/o)
- Having children or dependents other than a spouse
- Handicap or other disability

On the other hand, the term low GPA applicant may not be as straightforward as you would think. Yes, as the name suggests, people who fall into this category have a GPA that is less than ideal. While some may think that this means any GPA that is less than a 3.0, due to the competitive nature of the PA school application process, even those with GPAs between 3.0-3.49 are considered "low GPA" by some programs. Don't let this discourage you, though! Hang in there with me… I'm going to explain why.

I think it is important to point out that there are a few types of low GPA applicants. To help you understand, let me provide an example of each:

- **Student A**: Did not do so well in the early semesters of college, but was able to change their grades around at some point. Although their overall GPA may still be low, their transcript reflects a consistent upward trend in grades.
- **Student B**: Had some semesters where they did extremely well, and others where they did not. Their transcript is a mix of high and low grades spread throughout their college career.
- **Student C**: Had a rough time throughout college and was never really able to adjust or perform well. Their transcript reflects grades that are consistently average to below average, especially in the sciences.

My undergraduate academic journey had aspects of students A, B, and C above. Because of this, I had to work ten times harder than the typical applicant. Being able to identify and understand what type of applicant you are will help you better strategize how you can make yourself a competitive applicant to PA school, in spite of any academic shortcomings.

My Personal Experience With This

When I first decided to apply to PA school in 2014, I was not yet aware that I was a low GPA applicant. After being academically dismissed from college in 2007, I took a four-year hiatus in my education. When I felt like I could once again focus on my studies, I enrolled at a new university as a sophomore biology major. I did fairly well in school this time around and worked hard to maintain my GPA at a 3.0+. Finally, in the spring semester of 2014, my long and winding journey with college came to an end, and I received a bachelor's degree in biology.

I knew that I was a non-traditional applicant because I had a large gap in my undergraduate education and I was an older student. However, because I graduated with a 3.0, I did not classify myself as a low GPA applicant to PA school. It wasn't until after I was rejected from every single program I applied to that first cycle that I realized my GPA was not competitive at all.

What went wrong? Several things actually. For one, I didn't have any healthcare experience when I applied the first time. Although the programs I applied to back then didn't *require* it, they did *strongly suggest* applicants have some background experience in patient care, but I chose to ignore this and take my chances. However, the bigger issue was, I lacked the understanding of how my GPA was being calculated and assessed by both CASPA and PA programs. To this day, I still shake my head when I think back to how unprepared I was during that first application cycle.

Having a good understanding of how programs will review your overall application is essential to making sure you understand where you stand in terms of competitiveness. Without this, it will be very difficult for you to formulate a plan or strategy to apply if you are a non-traditional and/or low GPA applicant. In the next chapter, I'll discuss the application process, including GPA categories, how they are calculated, and why this is important.

CHAPTER 3:
UNDERSTANDING THE CASPA GPA CALCULATION PROCESS

I could have saved myself a lot of heartache my first application cycle had I just been aware of the information in this chapter.

The Centralized Application Service for Physician Assistants, otherwise known as CASPA is the online application portal for all those interested in applying to PA school. It allows applicants to apply to multiple accredited PA programs located in the U.S. through just one application. The majority of PA programs utilize CASPA to streamline their application process. However, be aware that there are a few schools that do not use CASPA, and instead require applicants to submit applications to them directly.

CASPA operates on a cyclical basis. It opens up in April of each year, typically on the last Thursday of the month, and concludes on April 1st of the following year. Once CASPA opens, applicants are then able to create an account (if it is their first time applying) and select which programs they want to submit applications to. The CASPA website lists all the PA programs that participate within their system, including their respective deadlines. Before you can submit your application, you will need to upload all the necessary materials and pay the application fee. Once this is done, your application will undergo a verification process which can take anywhere from a few days to a few weeks. CASPA will notify you when verification is complete, and will then forward your application to the programs you selected.

The Verification Process

As a low GPA applicant, the CASPA verification process is something that can either make or break you. Having an understanding of how verification works, as well as what information schools will have access to, will better help you determine your readiness to apply.

So, what is verification? From the CASPA website:

> *Verification is the process used to ensure all of your coursework was entered correctly and consistently. Since credit values, grade values, and course subjects vary widely from school to school, your programs need some type of standardization so they can accurately compare applicants. This standardization is achieved by using your coursework to* ***create a standard set of GPAs****, ensuring you are compared to other applicants fairly and equally.*

To help you further understand, all applicants are required to enter all coursework and grades received from every college or university attended, whether you graduated from there or not. In addition to this, CASPA requires you to forward your transcripts from every college or university attended so they can verify the information you entered for accuracy. After your transcripts are received, they will begin their verification process and the end result will be a set of GPAs calculated by their standards. This set of GPAs are what PA programs will utilize in their review process, unless they state otherwise.[3]

I want to point out two very important things to understand about the verification process:

1. You are required to input ALL GRADES received for ALL COURSES taken. This means even the courses where you received letter grades of F (fail), WF (withdraw failing), W (withdraw), I (incomplete), and NC (no credit).
2. CASPA DOES NOT honor grade forgiveness and therefore factors in all grades received from all attempts in their GPA calculations. What this means is if you retook a class for a higher grade, and your school replaced the lower grade with the higher grade, CASPA will still factor in BOTH grades when they compute your GPA if both grades appear on your transcript.

I have found that a lack of understanding of the above two points, as well as misconceptions about the CASPA GPA calculations is where most low GPA PA school applicants go wrong, including myself.

My Personal Experience With This

I first applied to PA school the semester before I completed my bachelor's degree in biology. By that point, I had already attended four universities and needed to forward all four transcripts to CASPA.

Just to give you some background history, I began my freshman year of college as a biology major at C.W. Post Long Island University, and transferred to Stony Brook

[3] More on this topic in Chapter 8 of this book.

University after two semesters. Unfortunately, my time at Stony Brook was affected by personal issues that led to me being depressed and unable to focus on my classes. Because of this, I was placed on academic suspension for having a GPA less than a 2.0 after three consecutive semesters, which meant that I could not take classes at Stony Brook that following semester, and would need to petition to be reinstated.

In hindsight, I should have taken some time off school so that I could regain my focus, but I was still in denial at this point. So instead, I enrolled in four classes at Nassau Community College: two sciences (Microbiology and General Chemistry 2), and an English and history course. At the end of this semester, my GPA was a 2.39 after receiving three Bs and one F (I failed General Chemistry 2), but I still went ahead and petitioned to be readmitted to Stony Brook and was somehow granted conditional reinstatement. The terms of my reinstatement required that I maintain a GPA above 2.0 in the semester of my reinstatement. Unfortunately, I did not meet this criteria as my GPA fell to a 0.93, the lowest it had ever been. As such, I was academically dismissed from Stony Brook, having earned barely enough credits to be considered a sophomore.

I had no choice but to take time off from my education as no college would accept me with such a low GPA. In the interim, I took the time to work on myself and reassess what I wanted out of life. Even though I knew it would be hard to get back into school, I did not want to give up on my dream of practicing medicine. Fortunately, I was able to connect with a gentleman who held a high position in school administration and who believed in my potential. Through his connections, I was able to return to college nearly four years after my dismissal from Stony

Brook. I finished my sophomore, junior, and senior years of undergrad at CUNY City College of NY and was proud to have maintained a 3.0 GPA throughout my remaining semesters.

So here's where I made my first mistake. Because I had done well at CUNY City College of NY and graduated with a 3.0 GPA, I thought *this* GPA would be the one PA programs would review, since this was the college I earned my bachelor's degree from.

My second mistake was not being aware that ALL the grades from EVERY course I ever took at EVERY single college I attended would be utilized in the CASPA verification process to generate my GPA. My third mistake was not realizing that CASPA generates several different GPAs at the end of their verification process, and *these* GPAs are primarily what PA programs utilize when they review applications to see if applicants meet their admissions criteria.

You can imagine my surprise and shock when I saw that my cumulative undergraduate GPA was a 2.27, as calculated by CASPA at the end of my verification process. This was because although I had done well at City College of NY, my previous failing grades overshadowed all of this, and tanked my GPA to below what is considered competitive for all of the PA schools on my list. Needless to say, I was rejected from every program I applied to that first cycle.

After a bit of research, I understood where I went wrong and enrolled in both post-baccalaureate and graduate courses after that first cycle, therefore adding two more universities to my long list of schools attended, and two more transcripts for CASPA to review as part of their verification. Because I did well in those courses, my GPA rose a bit higher my second cycle applying, and even higher my third and final cycle when I was finally accepted to PA school. In Part 2 of this book, I go into further detail about how I was able to raise my GPA and make myself a competitive applicant.

The Different CASPA GPA Categories

The Transcript Entry section of CASPA is where you will input all your courses and the grades received in them. For each course entered, you will need to select from a standardized list of course subjects that is generated by CASPA in conjunction with PAEA. These course subjects fall into several categories that CASPA will use to calculate several types of GPAs. (It is important to familiarize yourself with the course subjects and what classes fall under each category. To do so, please visit the CASPA website, or enter "CASPA Course Subject List" in your search engine box).

The CASPA GPA types are as follows:

- Year-Level GPAs→ CASPA calculates a GPA for each academic year of college (freshman, sophomore, junior, and senior), as well as post-baccalaureate and graduate coursework, if applicable. (See Appendix B for my year level GPA breakdown.)
- Course Subject Category GPAs→ All the courses you took will be categorized under the following subject headings: Biology/Zoology, Inorganic Chemistry, Organic Chemistry, Biochemistry, Physics, Other Science, Math, English, Behavioral Science, and Other Non-Science. A GPA for each of these subjects will be generated. Please note, a BCP GPA will also be generated and is comprised

of courses that fall under the subjects of Biology, Chemistry, and/or Physics.

- Science and Non-Science GPAs→ This GPA type is a further breakdown of the two above. The Year-Level GPAs are further divided into Science, Non-Science, and Overall/Total (science plus non-science) using the course subject headings above.

Each of these GPA types are displayed as part of the Academic History section of your CASPA, and are able to be viewed by PA programs. The GPA requirement for each PA program may vary, however, in my experience, the GPAs most commonly utilized by programs are the cumulative undergraduate GPA as well as the science GPA as determined by CASPA. These are also the GPAs that tend to hinder most low GPA applicants from applying to PA school.

But don't worry, this book will guide you on how to overcome this setback and move forward with pursuing your dream of becoming a PA.

Other Important Things to Know and Remember

One question that I get asked frequently is how W letter grades affect your chances of applying to PA school. Keep in mind, a W means that you withdrew from a class without penalty. This is different from a WF, which means you withdrew from a class because you were failing. CASPA will count WF grades as part of their GPA calculations, but W grades are not factored in and have no impact on your GPA.

HOWEVER...

Because you need to input all courses taken, as well as grades received on CASPA, PA programs are able to see any course that you received a W in. Depending on how many Ws you received, programs may question why you had to withdraw from a course or courses, and this may raise some concern as to the reasons why you were unable to complete the course. For example, were you inefficient at studying, are you unable to handle a full-time course load, or was there a personal issue?

A W grade is still better than an F, so my advice is if you feel like you are in jeopardy of failing, it is better to withdraw from a course before that happens. However, try to limit the number of times you withdraw from a class, especially if it is a science course. If you happen to have several Ws on your transcript, this may be something you need to explain in your personal statement. Chapter 9 of this book has all the information you need regarding writing your personal statement as well as how to address any issues that may be seen as a red flag.

Another thing to note is that non-CASPA PA programs will have their own way of standardizing GPAs. Because of this, it would be wise for you to check with them directly regarding their admissions criteria and requirements.

Lastly, you do not necessarily need to wait for the CASPA verification process to have an idea of what your GPA will be. The CASPA website has more information on how your credit hours are converted to generate a GPA if you would like to manually calculate your GPA. Their website also has a link to a GPA calculator you can utilize, however, there are also several other online GPA calculators that can also help you determine your GPA.

Part 2:

Exploring Your 'GPA Fix' Options

Chapter 4:
Completing your Bachelor's Degree

Note: The information in this chapter is geared toward those who are in the process of completing their first bachelor's degree. If you have already completed your degree, then you may find it more helpful to skip·ahead to the next chapter.

In my years of mentoring 'low GPA' pre-PA students, I have come to learn that those who have not yet achieved their bachelor's degree and have concerns about applying to PA school fall into the following categories:

- Started undergrad at some point, but are not currently enrolled
- Currently enrolled as an undergrad student and have earned a few bad grades here and there
- Nearing the final semester of undergrad (90+ credits) and will be graduating with a low science and/or low overall GPA

I understand that there are a myriad of reasons why the above categories may apply to you. In my case, the struggles I was experiencing in my personal life were affecting my ability to concentrate on my studies. Perhaps your reasons may be dealing with medical problems, a family situation, or financial issues. No matter what the reasons are, it is important that once you make the decision to pursue the PA career path, you do whatever is necessary to make sure you complete your bachelor's degree and FINISH STRONG, regardless of which of these categories you fall under.

Here are a few things for you to consider:

NOT CURRENTLY ENROLLED?

Whether you have chosen to take a break from school, are suspended, or have been dismissed, you need to work on a plan to get yourself back into school. Remember, obtaining a bachelor's degree is an **absolute** requirement for PA school.

When considering your return, make sure you assess and analyze the reasoning behind why you are not currently enrolled. For example, did you have to work full-time to support yourself and couldn't handle being a full-time student at the same time? If so, what changes will you make to ensure that this will not affect your studies once you re-enroll?

Ask yourself the following questions:

1. *Do you need to change your major?*[4]
2. *Should you start over at a new university or college?*
3. *Should you consider part-time vs full-time enrollment?*
4. *Are you or can you be fully committed to your studies at this present time?*

The idea behind asking yourself the above questions is that taking a leave of absence from school is something

[4] Remember, you do not need to have a specific major for PA school admissions as long as you can complete the prerequisite courses and other requirements.

you will more than likely need to address in your PA school application or PA school interview. It will have a less damaging effect on your application if you are able to demonstrate improvement from the point you returned to school **through** the time of completing your bachelor's. It is imperative that you make the necessary decisions and changes that will enable you to be successful.

But please → Be realistic with yourself and take the time to really evaluate if your current circumstances allow you to commit to school once again.

ENROLLED, BUT WORRIED ABOUT BAD GRADES?

Whether you have had a bad semester(s), or have a few Cs, Ds, or Fs sprinkled here and there, what is most important is that you do your best to rectify the situation. If possible, retake the course for a higher grade. If you are still early on in your undergraduate career and have not yet taken that many credits (think less than 60), this may not affect your final GPA quite as much, if you can pull yourself together and demonstrate an upward trend. A few bad grades are not the end of the world, even if they are in science or PA prerequisite courses.

You also may want to consider changing your major from science to non-science, if it will keep you from causing further damage to your GPA. For example, if you are a chemistry major, but find you are struggling with the courses that are mandatory for you take in your major, you can switch to a psychology major and just plan to take the prerequisite courses along the way, or after you complete your undergrad (more on this in the next chapters). Being a science major definitely has its benefits, one being that it makes completing the PA school prerequisite courses much easier, since chances are some of those courses will be required for your Bachelor of Science degree. However, as a reminder, PA programs DO NOT require you to have a specific major or degree in order to apply (as long as you complete the prerequisites).

If you are close to graduating, and have several semesters of bad or failing grades, you may have noticed that the more credits you earn, the less your GPA will budge. In this case, do your best to finish strong anyway, and read on to the next chapters to find out what you can do to mitigate this.

"You cannot change the past, but you can make the changes necessary to keep it from affecting your future."

Chapter 5: Post-Baccalaureate Studies

My "informal post-bacc" further helped me establish the upward academic trend that PA programs look favorably upon when considering low GPA applicants.

So, What Is a Post-Baccalaureate?

In short, a post-baccalaureate or post-bacc as it is most commonly referred to, is any coursework, program of study, or academic research that is obtained **AFTER** a bachelor's degree but **BEFORE** obtaining a graduate degree.

There are two main reasons why people choose to pursue a post-bacc:

1. *To take prerequisite courses required for graduate level programs*
2. *To enhance or strengthen their current academic record*

For those of us "with low GPAs", one or both of the above reasons may apply to your situation. For example, perhaps you started off as a non-science major or switched from a science major to non-science major at some point during undergrad and still need to complete the PA school prerequisites. If that is the case, then a post-bacc is for you! Or perhaps you are someone who struggled in the sciences during undergrad for whatever underlying reason, but you are confident that you can make the cut and want a second chance to prove it. Again, then a post-bacc is for you!

Why Should You Consider a Post-bacc?

Common Misconception:

Once you graduate with your bachelor's degree, you cannot change your cumulative undergraduate GPA. Ever.

When you finally graduate from college or university, your final transcript will list your cumulative undergraduate GPA for all grades earned towards your bachelor's degree. When people reach out to me, it is usually this GPA that they are worried about, or feel that they are doomed to live with forever, and rightfully so. Any quick search on Google about "How to get into PA school" will undoubtedly say that a high cumulative GPA is needed. But what is important to note, and what most people don't understand, is:

You Can Change Your Cumulative Undergraduate GPA.

Yup. Read that bolded and underlined sentence again. This point is especially true as it pertains to applying to PA school, and the reason is based on how CASPA will factor in post-bacc courses into their GPA calculations.

How CASPA Factors in a Post-bacc

In Chapter 3, I broke down the CASPA GPA application process and the many different factors that come into play when they calculate your GPA on behalf of PA programs.

There are several GPA types that CASPA calculates and breaks down on the 'Academic History' portion of your CASPA application. The GPA types are as follows:

- Year-Level GPAs
- Course Subject Category GPAs
- Science and Non-Science GPAs

The first GPA type: Year-Level GPAs are what those applying to PA school with low GPAs should be most grateful for because it allows for us to have a "second chance." This GPA type will break down your GPA for each academic year of undergrad: Freshman, Sophomore, Junior, and Senior year. BUT if you are someone who has completed a post-bacc, they will then combine your post-bacc coursework as part of their cumulative undergraduate GPA calculation.[5] Let that sink in!

In case it isn't clear to you yet, this means that if you choose to do a post-bacc, any course that you take as part of this post-bacc will give you the opportunity to **raise your cumulative undergraduate GPA** and therefore become a more competitive applicant, in spite of your past academic history.

Before you get to celebrating, arm yourself with the knowledge of how to do a post-bacc, and my experience with this.

---

[5] From the CASPA website: Using Quality Points, CASPA calculates a GPA for each academic year. GPAs from your Freshman, Sophomore, Junior, and Senior academic years are subsequently:

1. Combined with any post-baccalaureate coursework to create a cumulative undergraduate GPA, and
2. Combined with any post-baccalaureate coursework plus any graduate coursework to create an overall GPA.

The Different Types of Post-baccs

While the information in this chapter may or may not have been known to you prior to reading this, I can assure you that the method of doing a post-bacc is commonly known to most large institutions, as many have started to capitalize on this. If there is one thing I want to make sure you clearly understand, it is the following:

You do not need to enroll in a formal post-bacc program in order to complete a post-bacc.

As a reminder, a post-bacc is any and all courses taken after earning your bachelor's degree but before your graduate degree. Keeping this in mind, if you choose to take a couple of courses at your local university or college post-undergrad, this would be considered a post-bacc.

There are two ways to do a post-bacc, which I have playfully called: the 'Do it Their Way' (DITW) and the 'Do it Your Way' (DIYW):

1. **DITW:** Enrolling in a formal (structured) post-bacc program affiliated with a college or university.
2. **DIYW:** Not enrolling in a formal post-bacc program and taking courses *at will* (unstructured) at a college or university.

Out of both of these options,
I highly recommend option #2: DIYW.

I have noticed over the years of my coaching pre-PA students that there have been several pre-health post-bacc programs offered through colleges and universities, many of them targeting pre-med and pre-PA students. While in theory there is nothing wrong with this, the problem is that many, if not all, of these programs that fall under the DITW category come at a hefty tuition price. And because they are post-bacc programs, many students are not able to utilize financial aid or grants to cover these expensive costs, and instead try to find a way to foot the bill via private loans.

The main reason I preach NOT going this route is because there are no real benefits to taking the formal route versus taking the informal route. Unlike some of the formal post-bacc programs offered to pre-med students, doing a formal (DITW) post-bacc and completing it successfully will not guarantee you an interview or a direct admission to a PA program. So while it is convenient to go this route because most of them will bundle courses for you, in my opinion, you are much better off completing a DIYW post-bacc.

One of the major benefits of a DIYW, besides the lower cost, is the fact that you are free to take the courses you feel you need or will offer the most benefit to you. For example, I am someone who did horrible in chemistry and needed to utilize lots of resources just to get a passing grade.[6] On the other hand, I loved my biology courses, and found them easier to study and understand on my own.

During my post-bacc, I chose not to give myself the added stress of taking chemistry courses, and focused primarily on biology-based courses (although I did take Biochemistry but found this much more feasible than General or Organic Chemistry). This is something I would not have been able to do if I enrolled in a formal (DITW) post-bacc program. Since they have a curriculum already

---

[6] To this day, just reading or hearing the word chemistry puts me on edge.

built out for you, you have no choice but to take the courses assigned within their time frame and schedule.

My Personal Experience With This

I began my DIYW post-bacc a semester after I graduated with my bachelor's degree. I had previously applied to PA school (my first cycle applying), and had started to receive rejections, most providing me with the advice that my GPA was much too low to be considered and I needed to work on improving that. After doing my own research, I came across the option of doing a post-bacc. After understanding how CASPA would factor in a post-bacc, and deciding to go the DIYW route, I enrolled at a local college and estimated I would need approximately 35-40 credits of sciences to really make myself a competitive applicant. My GPA, that first cycle of applying, was a mere 2.27 and definitely not competitive enough.

It took me about 1.5 years to complete the 39 credits I ultimately earned, at full-time status, making sure I took a minimum of three courses a semester. In the end, I saved a lot of money, took classes that both fit my schedule and balanced each other well, and was able to earn all As and Bs because I was confident in the courses that I chose.

See Appendix C in the back of this book which lists the courses I took during my post-bacc. You should use this list as an example of courses you may want to *consider* taking, rather than a list of courses you absolutely have to take. Remember, the advantage of a DIYW is that you get to choose which courses you think will work in your favor.

In Chapter 7, you will find a sample list of courses that are commonly labeled as "suggested" or "recommended" courses for prospective applicants to PA school.

Some things to note when completing a post-bacc:

1. Make sure to take courses that you feel you will best succeed in
2. If possible, complete the **majority** of your courses at a 4-year university instead of a community college
3. Be sure to take at a minimum two courses at a time
4. It is best to enroll in 300-400 level science courses, as these are typically considered more difficult
5. You can complete post-bacc courses at more than one college or university if necessary
6. Talk to the financial aid office to see if you could benefit from enrolling as a non-matriculated versus matriculated (second bachelor's degree) student

A note on choosing to matriculate as a second bachelor's degree student (#6 above): This is an option that works best for those who still have remaining undergraduate financial aid monies or loans available to them. It is important to know that going this route does not mean you have to *actually* complete the second degree for the major you declare (obviously, it would be in your best interest to declare a science major). The idea is, you are simply using the second degree status as a strategy that will allow you to take the courses you need at a reduced cost—if you have undergraduate funds remaining.

Once you complete those courses, you can stop there and do not need to take whatever courses are remaining for that degree if they do not serve your purpose. Think of it as a sort of DIYW hack. As I mentioned above, the first step would be to talk to the financial aid office to see if this is even a feasible option for you. If it is, you may still want to compare the flexibility of taking courses via this option as opposed to enrolling as a non-matriculated (non-degree seeking) student.

CHAPTER 6: GRADUATE STUDIES

I pursued a Master of Public Health (MPH) as a backup plan. I figured, if I never got into PA school, at least I could still work in healthcare. And if I did get into PA school, the MPH would pair well with my PA training and allow me to enhance the quality of care I provide to my patients.

So What Falls Under Graduate Studies?

Courses taken either individually at the graduate level or within a graduate level program of study are considered graduate studies. To help make this point even clearer, let me provide you with three examples from my own pre-PA journey.

Example 1:

During undergrad, I had the opportunity to take an immunology course that was typically open to the Master's of Science students only, however the university was trying something new for those undergraduate students who wanted to challenge themselves. This immunology course was listed both on my transcript and on CASPA as a graduate course.

Example 2:

When I decided to enroll in an MPH (Master of Public Health) degree program, all the courses I took as part of this were listed on CASPA as 'Graduate.'

Example 3:

Before I was accepted into the MPH, I first decided to do a one semester certificate in a public health program. The courses that were a part of this certificate program were the same five courses that were a part of the first semester of the MPH, and were therefore considered graduate level coursework. This certificate program offered students the chance to see what an MPH course of study would be like. If you maintained a B+ average, then you were able to matriculate as an official MPH student (which is exactly what I ended up doing).

In case my point in the above examples is lost on you, what I want to make clear is that just like a post-bacc, you have a few options to choose from in deciding how to complete graduate studies. You can either take graduate level courses outside of an official degree or certificate granting program (like a DIYW post-bacc), OR you can enroll in a traditional master's degree or graduate level certificate program.

Why Should You Consider Graduate Studies?

Enrolling in graduate courses is a good option if you find yourself in the following situations:

1. You have already completed a post-bacc in the past, but your cumulative undergraduate GPA is still not competitive enough
2. It is more cost-effective for you to take out graduate loans (or graduate financial aid) to finance your post-undergraduate coursework
3. You are interested in a particular graduate degree or graduate certificate that you think would enhance your future career goals as a PA

How CASPA Factors In Graduate Courses

In the previous chapter, I broke down how the CASPA GPA calculation works to the benefit of those who are considering a post-bacc.

As a recap, there are several GPA types that CASPA factors into their GPA calculation and include as part of the Academic History portion of your CASPA application. The GPA types are as follows:

- Year-Level GPAs
- Course Subject Category GPAs
- Science and Non-Science GPAs

The first type: Year-Level GPAs, will include the courses you took each year during undergrad. However, it will also list any courses you took as a post-bacc and/or graduate student as well.

Why is this important? Well, in the previous chapter, I mentioned the cumulative undergraduate GPA that CASPA calculates consists of all undergraduate courses **PLUS** any post-bacc courses. However, the overall GPA calculation factors in all undergraduate courses, post-bacc courses **PLUS** any graduate courses you have taken.

Below is a chart that may simplify what I have said above.

Year-Level GPA Breakdown

Year	Description
Freshman	Freshman year GPA
Sophomore	Sophomore year GPA
Junior	Junior year GPA
Senior	Senior year GPA

Total	Freshman + Sophomore + Junior + Senior years GPA
Post-Baccalaureate	Sum of GPA of Post-bacc
Cumulative Undergraduate	Total +/- Post-bacc GPA*
Graduate	Sum of GPA of Graduate courses
Overall	Total Cumulative Undergraduate +/- Graduate GPA*

Please Note: The +/- indicated on the chart above is dependent on whether or not you took post-bacc and/or graduate courses

Every PA program has different requirements when it comes to their GPA minimums. This is precisely why CASPA breaks it down into several different GPA types. In my experience, the majority of PA programs have a minimum requirement for cumulative undergraduate GPA, overall GPA, science GPA, or any combination of the three. This is why your strategy should be to aim for the highest GPA possible in all categories given your circumstance.

My Personal Experience With This

If I'm being completely honest, the sole reason why I chose to enroll in graduate studies is because I was starting to lose hope that I would ever get into PA school. When I applied to PA schools for the second time around, I had completed one full semester of a post-bacc, was in the middle of completing another one, AND I had just started a certificate in a public health graduate program.[7] In hindsight, because my GPA was so low to begin with, I probably should have waited to apply again until I had completed more courses so that I could really show PA programs that I was capable of exceeding in science courses. However, I was eager to apply and wanted to see if I would "get lucky" this time around. When I was rejected by yet another CASPA cycle, my confidence started to slip a little.

Being that I am a practical person, and also try to plan every detail of my life, I figured the smart (safe) thing to do would be to have a Plan B. Actually, I guess it was more like Plan C because Plan B was doing a post-bacc. I knew I still wanted to work in the healthcare field in some capacity, and I had always found public health to be interesting. As a future PA, I had plans to work on implementing community health interventions within underserved communities both locally and internationally. I figured if I eventually got into PA school, the MPH would be a great degree to have as well because of my future goals. And if I never got into PA school, I could still work to improve the health of others as a public health professional. That was my Plan B/C.

What I did not know at the time, and would find out later during my PA school interviews, is that PA schools were actually more impressed with my post-bacc coursework since the courses were a more accurate reflection of my capability of handling difficult science and medical-based coursework. You see, the MPH curriculum typically does not include courses that fall

---

[7] Yep. I was enrolled in both undergraduate and graduate courses simultaneously because I was eager to get into PA school and didn't want to "waste" any more time. Between classes, full-time work, and a part-time job, I was sleep deprived that year.

under the science designation and since I had done so poorly in the sciences for the first half of undergrad, it was imperative that I show programs I could excel in the sciences.

I am not sharing my experience with graduate school to discourage or even encourage you to blindly follow in my footsteps. To this day, I have yet to meet another pre-PA who is in as bad shape as I was. As a reminder, I was an applicant who was once academically dismissed from undergrad because my GPA fell below a 1.0. I worked hard to get myself into PA school, but realistically, I needed to have a backup plan because of the damage I did to my academic history. You may not necessarily need to pursue a whole other degree as a backup plan, but that choice is ultimately up to you and whatever you are most comfortable with.

If you are still undecided as to whether or not you should do a post-bacc, graduate, or both, read on to the next chapter, where I provide you with additional details that may help make your decision easier.

CHAPTER 7: DETERMINING WHICH 'GPA FIX' IS BEST FOR YOU

My pre-PA journey could be summed up by 4 Ps: Plan, Persistence, Patience, and Perseverance.

So how do you decide if you should do a post-bacc, graduate coursework, or both? Well, the answer really depends on your specific situation. I have been mentoring low GPA pre-PAs long enough to know that there are several factors you may need to consider in order to determine which option works best for you.

Post-bacc Route

This may be the best option if you are someone who:

- ➢ Needs to take (or retake) the PA prerequisite courses
- ➢ May benefit from taking additional science courses to boost your science GPA and/or make your application more competitive
- ➢ Did not major in the sciences during undergrad
- ➢ Can tap into remaining undergraduate financial aid and declare a second bachelor's degree

Pros:

- ❑ In DIYW post-bacc, you have the flexibility to choose your courses, working at your pace and with your schedule

- ❑ In DITW post-bacc, there is variation in curriculum with a high emphasis on science or medical-based courses
- ❑ Typically more affordable than a graduate degree (especially DIYW)

Cons:

- ❑ May have to pay out of pocket as classes may not be covered by financial aid or private student loans
- ❑ If you have already taken a lot of science courses during undergrad, there may be very few courses remaining for you to choose from

Graduate Studies Route

May be the best option if you are someone who:

- ➢ Has already completed a post-bacc but did not do as well as you would have liked
- ➢ Would like to pursue a graduate degree or graduate certificate program as an interest or backup plan
- ➢ Is an older student or career changer and do not prefer to take courses with undergraduate students
- ➢ Finds it easier to utilize graduate school loans and financial aid instead of paying out of pocket for a post-bacc

Pros:

- ❑ Courses offered tend to favor full-time work schedules
- ❑ Increased availability of online courses
- ❑ Can make you more marketable in your future career
- ❑ Ability to tap into graduate financial aid, grants, and loans

Cons:

- ❑ Can decrease the availability of graduate loan monies when it comes time to finance your PA education
- ❑ Additional student loan debt
- ❑ 1-2 year commitment

Other Important Things to Keep in Mind

Whichever option you choose, it is important that you make sure you are committed to doing what it takes to pull in the high grades/GPA you will need to make the difference in your PA school applications. PA programs can be forgiving of a low undergrad GPA if you can demonstrate an upward trend in your post-undergrad coursework.

Before you embark on either route, you will need to determine approximately how many credits or courses you will need to take to achieve a desirable GPA. You can do this by utilizing any online GPA calculator. Before you take on additional courses, I always advise that you first start with the PA school prerequisites. If you have grades of C or less in more than two of these required courses, then it would be wise for you to retake them as these courses are usually what PA program admissions utilize to determine eligibility for interview. From there, you can choose to take on additional coursework to make your application more competitive.

Courses To Consider

In terms of courses, your goal should be to take primarily science courses (especially if your science GPA is low), followed by health or medical related coursework during either your post-bacc or master's.

Some examples of common courses you should consider beyond the prerequisites are:

Science

Advanced Physiology
Analytical Chemistry
Biochemistry
Cell Biology
Developmental Biology
Embryology
Endocrinology
Genetics
Histology
Immunology
Molecular Biology
Neurobiology
Neurology
Organic Chemistry
Pathology
Pathophysiology
Pharmacology
Physics
Virology

Other

Abnormal Psychology
Medical Ethics

First Aid and CPR
Health Psychology
Life Span Psychology (aka Developmental Psychology)
Medical Terminology
Nutrition

Most of the above courses are listed on PA program websites as "suggested" or "highly recommended" courses, so it would be in your best benefit to take some of these, even if they are not listed as a prerequisite course for admission.

You should take a MINIMUM of two courses at a time (6-8 credits), but if you are able to take three or more, that is even better. Why is that? Remember, your goal, as a low GPA applicant, is to show PA program admissions that you are capable of handling difficult coursework. Anyone can take one course during a semester and get an A in it. But can you take 2-4 difficult sciences and get an A? This is what the program administration will be looking for in determining your capability as a future PA student. Additionally, the more classes you can take a semester, the sooner you can apply with confidence. But don't rush or push yourself! Choose your classes wisely and be sure to balance the harder courses with the easier ones to ensure your success. Remember, your ultimate goal is to establish an upward trend in grades and increase your GPA.

Academics are a huge part of your PA school application and an important part of your future success as a PA student. Although you've made some mistakes in the past, as long as you are focused, determined, and committed to putting in the hard work, you can become a competitive applicant to PA school. If becoming a PA is your dream career, keep your head down, come up with a plan, and get to work. Time will pass anyway... wouldn't you rather spend it doing the things that can help you accomplish your goals?

Part 3:

Beyond Academics

Chapter 8: Identify and Select PA Programs That Are the Best Fit

---

This is probably the most important chapter of the whole book.

Why? Because after all your hard work of taking more classes, acing those classes, increasing your patient care experience, and building connections you have finally, finally, FINALLY reached a point where you are ready to start compiling a list of PA schools you can apply to.

This is also usually the point where students reach out to me in desperation because they are confused as to where to begin, what to look for, or are discouraged when they research schools only to see PA program after program list that "their most competitive applicants have a GPA of 3.5+." This can be disheartening, but the good news is, out of 277 PA programs, there are more than a handful that I assure you will give your application a fair chance. Programs such as these have alternative criteria for admissions, which tend to work in favor of applicants who may not meet the typical standard requirements.

I have found that the most confusing part of the process in all of this is what to look for in a PA program as a low GPA applicant. Whether you chose to do a post-bacc, second bachelor's degree, certificate program, or a master's degree, the courses you took have been able to help you establish an upward academic trend (assuming you earned nothing below a B in your courses). Unfortunately, even though you have done well in your most recent coursework, the bad grades you earned during undergrad will still come back to haunt you simply because:

CASPA GPA calculations do not honor grade forgiveness or replacement.

What this means is depending on how low your GPA was at the time you graduated from college, your cumulative and overall GPA may not have the significant increase you were hoping for, even after taking additional courses. This is the part that usually trips people up, and has them worried that they are not eligible to apply, or worse, that they may need to take a gazillion more credit hours. Pause, take a deep breath, and hear me when I say: You have options.

My Personal Experience With This

As I mentioned earlier in this book, my first cycle applying to PA schools was right after I completed my Bachelor's degree in Biology (after previously failing college). I was so eager to apply and move forward with my education that I failed to do the appropriate research. You see, because I graduated with a 3.0 GPA, I thought I was in the category of students who could apply to any program without worry. I chose eleven programs, all located on the East Coast, and sat back with confidence, thinking that at least half of those programs would want to accept a student like me. The crazy thing is, I didn't even flinch when I saw that CASPA calculated my cumulative GPA as a 2.27, and the majority of the programs on my list required a GPA of at least 3.0. I just assumed the PA programs I applied to would take note of how hard I worked since returning to school, and would ignore my past academic indiscretions.

Boy, was I wrong. The eleven rejections I received that first cycle showed me that I was highly mistaken. After doing extensive research, I realized what areas of my application I needed to improve. But more importantly, I recognized that I had applied to all the wrong schools!

When it came time for me to reapply to my second cycle of CASPA, I had done a bit more research and realized where I went wrong in that first cycle. I needed to target the PA programs I applied to and submit applications to only those programs that did not have set GPA requirements and/or programs that took a holistic approach when reviewing candidates. Once I figured this out, I had much better luck the second time I applied to PA schools. Even though I still received a couple of rejections, I was able to grab the attention of two programs and was invited to interview with them. In the end, I was waitlisted, but I still considered this to be a success because I made it to the interview phase of the application process.[8]

By the time I applied for that third and final CASPA cycle, I was a professional at picking which schools to apply to, and was glad to see that there were a few more options for applicants like me to choose from. At this point, I had also completed both my post-bacc and MPH, and had accrued plenty of varied patient care experience (PCE), so I was a much more competitive applicant

---

[8] After the PA school interview, a program will either accept you, reject you, or place you on their waitlist which means you are "on hold" until (hopefully), a seat opens up.

overall. This time, I was invited to three interviews and gained acceptance to TWO PA PROGRAMS.

If it were not for the fact that I researched each and every PA program to see which would be the best fit for me, I may not have ever received interviews, or worse yet, would have never been accepted to PA school.

I want to keep you from making the same mistakes I did, because applying to the wrong PA schools can be a very expensive mistake.

What Is Holistic Admissions?

As a non-traditional and/or low GPA applicant, you may have heard that the best schools for you to apply to are those that are considered "holistic." So how to find one? There are some PA program websites that identify as such, sometimes listing that they take a holistic approach to their admissions processes and application review. Other PA programs do not use this terminology at all, but their admissions criteria would qualify as holistic for all intents and purposes.

So what does the term *holistic* really mean? To put it simply, it means considering the "whole person" instead of just certain components. As it pertains to PA Admissions, this means your application as a whole would be considered to determine your eligibility as a student, not just your GPA, test scores, or whatever other negative items you may have on your application.

Programs that participate in holistic admissions factor in aspects of your application, such as your background, age, ethnicity, quality and type of patient care experience, letters of recommendation, extracurriculars, evidence of leadership, commitment to service, and unique experiences. This is why it is very important to also strengthen areas outside of academics, as well as tell your story in your personal statement and supplemental essays (more on this in Chapter 9).

I wish I could say finding programs such as these is as easy as Googling 'Holistic PA Schools.' While a few options may come up on a search, I can guarantee that there are far more programs that take this approach than may appear in your search. What is even more confusing is that even if a program does state that they are *holistic*, that may not necessarily mean that you fit their eligibility criteria. In fact, there are some programs that consider themselves to be holistic, but still require a high minimum GPA.

Another thing to keep in mind is that PA programs may change their admissions requirements from cycle to cycle, so just because they accepted or did not accept something last cycle, does not mean that may still be the case for the cycle you apply. As such, I always encourage applicants to stay up-to-date on a particular program of interest and their requirements, and do your own research instead of relying on the findings of another person.

For all these reasons above, I want to point out key factors you need to look out for when crafting your PA school list. This will help you identify programs whether you find success your first time applying, or need to reapply in subsequent cycles.

How to Craft Your PA School List

If I didn't make this clear in the above section, creating a list of PA schools that you are eligible to apply to will take quite a bit of research on your part. Quite often, I hear from applicants that they based their list on another applicant's research, or a list they found online on some blog or PA forum. While this may be helpful as a starting point, I strongly encourage you to do your own search, because the specifics of your application profile may not be the same as the next person.

Back when I was a prospective applicant, my main source of information came from PA program websites. But don't just look at the home page or admissions requirements section. Sometimes, the information I needed was on the FAQ page or in fine print under prerequisite courses. My point? ***Do thorough research.***

To help you move along faster in the process, here is one quick tip that could save you both some time and money:

---

*If a program states that they have a **REQUIRED** minimum GPA of ____________ and your GPA is less than that number, **DO NOT WASTE YOUR TIME APPLYING TO THAT SCHOOL**. I repeat, do not waste your time.*

This is the number one mistake I made during my first application cycle. The only exception to this rule is if that program also has a clause where they clearly state if/when they will allow GPAs that do not meet their posted minimum. I'd say more often than not, this exception, if it exists, will appear within the same section, so you won't have to dig too deep to find out whether or not you are eligible. If you do not see an exception listed, MOVE ON!!

Besides program websites, I also utilized PA program open houses, information sessions, or similar events to find out if an applicant like me would meet the criteria. Virtual or in-person PA program events are great opportunities for you to speak directly with PA program admissions personnel and find the answers you need. Lastly, if all else fails, do not hesitate to call a program directly or send an email. Sometimes this is the fastest option, depending on the time of year you are reaching out.[9] If you choose this method of contact, I always advise that you provide a little bit of background about who you are and your stats, including the upward academic trend you have been working hard to establish BEFORE you ask your questions. This can help the person you are corresponding with better understand if you do or do not fit what they are looking for in an applicant.

I would encourage you to apply broadly. While I firmly believe applicants like us have options, you have to be willing to step outside of your comfort zone, or more specifically, geographic location when it comes to PA school. The thing is, unlike someone with a perfect application profile, you do not have the luxury of being choosy when it comes to selecting schools. You can start with looking up programs in your state by utilizing a general directory such as the one found on the PAEA

---

[9] During peak application time, late April to approximately September of each year, PA programs are solely focused on admissions and may not respond promptly to general inquiries.

website,[10] or a simple internet search, but either way, you will need to branch out in order to find the schools where you fit best. As an added note, when you start your CASPA application, you will see a breakdown of all schools listed by state, so this is another helpful tool you can use. Keep in mind, there are some programs that do not use CASPA to accept applicants, but again, if you do your research, you will be able to find which programs do or do not.

Key Words, Phrases, and Tips

So what key things should you be looking for as you conduct your PA school research and work towards crafting an ideal PA program list for you?

I have broken it down by category below, and provided just a few examples of programs that fall under each category in Appendix D of this book to help you with this stage. This information is key to helping you determine which PA programs will acknowledge all the recent hard work you accomplished towards making yourself a competitive applicant.

Most Recent Credit Hours

When enrolling in courses either as a post-bacc or graduate student (as I discussed in Part 2 of this book), your goal is to establish an upward academic trend. By doing this, you will demonstrate to admissions that the poor grades you received earlier on in your education are not an accurate representation of your capabilities as a student.

---

10 PAEA stands for Physician Assistant Education Association and a list of PA programs in the U.S. can be found under their "Resources" tab.

PA programs will evaluate your performance in your most recent coursework to determine if you would be able to endure the rigorous PA school curriculum as a PA student. Programs that fall into this category will often specify the number of credit hours they will consider in their selection criteria. Typically, this is listed as the most recent 30, 40, or 60 credit hours taken. Oftentimes, the GPA for the most recent credits they require will also need to be at least a 3.0, although I have seen some programs allow as low as a 2.75.

3.0 in Completed Bachelor's Degree

When programs list this as part of their admissions requirement, what they are looking for specifically is the GPA you obtained at the university or college where you ultimately completed your bachelor's degree.

This is perfect if you are an applicant who began their undergraduate education at one school and did poorly, but transferred to another university where you successfully completed your bachelors with a GPA of 3.0 (similar to my story). If you were able to maintain an upward trend after you transferred, then you would be eligible for programs such as these.

On the flip side, if you are an applicant who has been able to establish an upward trend, but you remained at the same school throughout undergrad and your GPA unfortunately falls below the required minimum, then you are not an ideal applicant for programs that allow for this exception.

Replacement or Qualifying GPA

I love programs that do this! They really give the non-traditional students a chance. Keep in mind, they will still see your CASPA calculated GPA, however they will use your post-baccalaureate GPA, prerequisite GPA, or graduate degree GPA in their evaluation of your application. They will also specifically state which of these GPAs they will use and base their selection criteria on. Programs like this understand that mistakes can happen when you are a student, but if you are an applicant who has worked hard to improve upon their academics, then a program that allows for this GPA "switch" may work in your favor.

In fact, the PA program I attended had this as part of their admissions criteria. At the time I applied, they required a GPA of 3.0 in the prerequisite courses only (not overall). As long as your GPA for these seven courses was at or above a 3.0, then you met the eligibility requirement to apply. This is a perfect example of what I mean by a "qualifying GPA."

Admissions Appeal or Petition

Programs that have this as part of their admissions criteria are a blessing. Although they may list a required GPA, they will allow an exception for students who want to provide additional information that may help them understand the circumstances of why your GPA does not meet their criteria, and/or why you think in spite of this, you would be a great candidate for their PA program. This process of sending in additional documentation is known as a petition or appeal.

One thing to point out is even though this option is available for us low GPA applicants, you will need to have a *compelling* reason for your academic discrepancies. In addition to this, they will more than likely want you to provide proof that you are capable of succeeding as a PA student. The best way for you to do this? Establish an upward trend. If you need to, please go back and reread Part 2 (Chapters 4-7) of this book to review how and why.

GPA 2.75 cumulative and/or science GPA < 3.0

This is the most straightforward of all the categories listed. Programs that have a lower minimum GPA requirement for admissions recognize those of us who may have had a few academic hiccups along the way. They understand that this may have impacted your overall GPA, but does not necessarily mean you are a bad student; especially if you have done well in your most recent grades or were able to establish an upward trend.

If you have this minimum GPA straight out of undergrad, great. But this is also another way doing a post-bacc or graduate coursework will come in handy because the more classes you are able to take, the higher you will be able to raise your cumulative, overall, and/or science GPA.

Suggested, Recommended, or Preferred GPA or No GPA listed

I purposely saved this section for last because it is the most confusing of the options.

I am not going to lie to you. Programs that fall under this category are not my favorite because you are never really 100% sure you have a real chance. When I was applying, I emailed a few of these programs to find out if I was a good candidate. I received some lackadaisical and generic replies, such as: "You never know," or even, "Our program *may* consider your application." There was also the: "Our most competitive applicants have above a 3.0, but we don't have a set requirement" type of response.

Below is an actual email inquiry I sent to a program, as well as the response I received from the Director of Admissions a few days later.

1/21/22, 10:27 AM Gmail - PA applicant inquiry

Gmail Samora Charles <samora.charles@gmail.com>

PA applicant inquiry
4 messages

Samora Charles <samora.charles@gmail.com> Mon, Aug 1, 2016 at 6:16 AM
To: PAadmissions@ketchum.edu

Hello,

I am a prospective applicant to the PA program at Marshall B. Ketchum and I was wondering if I would be eligible to apply.

I received a BS in Biology in May 2013 and graduated with a 3.4 GPA. However, the earlier portion of my undergraduate career was not so great. Due to personal issues that impacted my grades heavily, I was academically dismissed from a university during my sophomore year of college-2007. Since then, I have done a science post-bacc, as well as 1 year of MPH courses all of which place my post-undergraduate GPA at 3.8.

I understand that this program recommends an overall cumulative GPA of 3.0 which I am sure I will not meet due to may past hardships. However my GPA for the listed prerequisites is above a 3.0. In addition, I have over 5 years of healthcare experience as a medical assistant and PCT, and scored a 158V and 155Q in my GRE.

Based on the above information, would my application be considered?

Any advice/guidance would be helpful,

Samora Charles

PA Admissions <paadmissions@ketchum.edu> Mon, Aug 1, 2016 at 6:12 PM
To: Samora Charles <samora.charles@gmail.com>

Hi Samora,

Thank you for your interest in our program.

No, you do not need to have a 3.0 GPA. You would still be eligible to apply to our program because a 3.0 is not *required* to apply. However, the most competitive applicants possess at a minimum an overall GPA of 3.0. With that said, MBKU is committed to conducting a "holistic" review of each individual application. This means we consider and take into account each aspect of the application when determining which applicants to invite for interviews.

To be eligible for review, all admissions requirements, degree and coursework prerequisites must be completed by the November 1st CASPA deadline.

I hope this helps. Please let me know if there's anything else I can assist you with.

https://mail.google.com/mail/u/0/?ik=4fdd95b035&view=pt&search=all&permthid=thread-f%3A1541455601060986935&simpl=msg-f%3A15414556010... 1/3

Success! As you can see, writing a detailed email providing them with a full picture may [hopefully] generate a detailed response from the program. This also works if you do happen to apply because you've now brought attention to your application. One PA program admin even wrote back to me saying "she would personally be looking out for my application!" This is why I always tell PA applicants ⇉ Call or Email programs if you have questions that can't be found on their website. It can ultimately work in your favor.

In Conclusion

The different categories I described above are the precise things I looked for as I researched PA programs to add to my list of PA schools I would be eligible to apply to. Had I been this strategic and meticulous my first time applying to PA school, I would have been able to save myself hundreds of dollars in wasted application fees.

Prior to applying the second time, I went through all 200+ PA programs listed on CASPA and searched their requirements, went through their FAQs, emailed or called admin if I was unclear if I met a requirement, and reached out to current students on social media, blogs, or forums. This did not take a few hours to do. I think it took a whole week to get through everything, and then additional time waiting to hear back about programs I was unsure of. But, in the end, I had generated a list of schools that I knew for sure would take an in-depth look at my application.

When you are at the point of creating a list, I recommend you reference this chapter again and again as you conduct your own research. You should use this as a guide as you comb through the different sections of PA program websites to see whether or not you meet their criteria. Remember, sometimes you may need to go beyond the large print on the home page or the Admissions Requirement section to find the answers you need, as demonstrated by some of the examples provided in Appendix D. You also need to remember that PA programs requirements may change from cycle to cycle, so if you have to reapply, you may need to adjust the list you created from the previous cycle to see if it still is accurate.

The research will take time, but be patient. The more programs you are able to confidently add to your list, the better your chances will be of getting into a school as a low GPA applicant. Remember, applying to PA school is not cheap, and rushing through this or not doing your due diligence can cost you your hard-earned money.

If I was able to accomplish this, and successfully, to get into PA school, so can you.

CHAPTER 9:
THE PERSONAL STATEMENT

Your personal statement should leave the reader with the impression that you have the personality, character, and background experience to succeed in PA school and beyond.

If academics and GPA is considered #1 on the list of important components of the pre-PA application to PA school, then I would say the personal statement, (often abbreviated as PS), is definitely #2. As a pre-PA mentor, I have read through dozens upon dozens of personal statements, and am passionate about making sure applicants understand that this is one area of the application you want to make sure you give the utmost attention and time to.

For us non-traditional, low GPA applicants, the personal statement is especially important because it is your opportunity to *tell your story* in your own words. Admissions will see your transcripts, GPA, scores etc. and may have already started to draw a conclusion as to whether or not you deserve an interview. But the personal statement is a tool you can use to get them to change their mind, or make them feel confident that you are someone they want to meet and should consider admitting to their program.

My Personal Experience With This

I consider myself to be a pretty decent writer. My love for writing is equally tied to my love of reading. As a child, I would read anything I could get my hands on, and even wrote my own short stories. One of my side hustles during high school and college was to revise and edit essays for any classmate that needed help. But when it came time to write my own personal statement for PA school, I found myself stuck and at a loss of where to begin. Each time I sat down to start writing, I would grapple with the question of how was I supposed to fit everything I wanted to say into a 5,000 character count essay? [11] It took several different drafts before I finally felt like I had written an essay that adequately described my motivation, my experiences, my setbacks, and why I felt like I should be given a chance. You can read a copy of my personal statement in Appendix E.

After I was accepted to PA school, I had the opportunity to ask a few of the faculty members who interviewed me why they decided to give me a chance. Most of them replied that although there were some concerns about my academics, my upward trend combined with my personal statement is what made them decide to at least offer me an interview so that they could get to know me beyond my application. After my interview, they were convinced that I had what it took to succeed as a PA student.

Own Your Story.

My point? Own your story. If you have done the hard work necessary to offset the negatives of your application, then you have no reason to be ashamed or try to hide the fact that you had some struggles along your pre-PA journey. Remember, the admissions department has access to your entire application, so there is no way for you to keep it a

[11] The CASPA personal statement has a 5,000 character limit which is equivalent to about 880 words or 1-1.5 pages.

secret. However, your words have the ability to tell them why you are more than the numbers listed on the GPA breakdown.

I was an applicant with a checkered academic past. I was embarrassed by how many Cs, Ds, and Fs were on my transcripts. I was even more embarrassed that I was academically dismissed from undergrad during my sophomore year. BUT I also knew how hard I later worked to change the narrative that I was a failure or a poor student. In my personal statement, I made sure to detail how I overcame all the obstacles that I faced, and how I persevered in spite of all the challenges. I used my failures as a strength. Your goal when writing your personal statement should be the same.

Writing Your Personal Statement

One of the biggest pieces of advice I like to share with those thinking of applying to PA school is to keep a journal or small notebook where you can jot down any memorable moments in either your personal or professional experiences that you feel have influenced your desire to pursue medicine, or more specifically become a PA. Within my personal statement, I chose to lead off with an experience I had while working as a patient care tech (PCT). It was a memory that solidified for me that there was no other career choice for me *but* to become a PA (see Appendix E).

By keeping track of any pertinent details, experiences, or memories that impacted you along your pre-PA journey, you will have created a resource that can help you when it comes time to draft your personal statement. If you haven't started this already, it is not too late to start. You can begin by reflecting back on your past experiences to see if anything stands out in your memory. If not, be sure to utilize this method moving forward for either recording experiences, ideas on what you may want to write about, quotes you identify with and why, or really anything that you think will help you get started with your writing.

I also want to point out that you should not feel like you have to have a single defining moment that led you down the path to PA. I read a lot of personal statements that include unnecessary dramatics, ill-placed quotes, or overly exaggerated statements all because you may have read or heard from someone else that these are items that help make your personal statement more interesting. This is not true at all, and including items that you *think* you need to have to fit the mold, can make your words come across as cliché and unoriginal. Your personal statement should be genuine and unique to **your background**.

I also urge applicants to get feedback on their personal statement *before* uploading it to their CASPA. This piece of advice applies to whether you think you are great at writing or are terrible at it. Your words may make sense to you, but how do they come across to outside readers? Even though I felt confident in my writing ability, I shared my personal statement with a few trusted individuals. By doing so, I was able to refine and revise my essay to a final product I was proud of.

Who should you get feedback from? In my opinion, the best people are either those who have some level of expertise in writing (think writing center at your school), or those who are familiar with the PA school application process (think PA students or working PAs). If you are able to have a combination of the two as readers, then that would be even better. However, I recommend receiving feedback from no more than three people max, as feedback is somewhat subjective, and having too many opinions can leave you frustrated and confused as you work towards a final draft. Utilize whatever free resources may already be within your reach, such as coworkers, PAs within your network, or mentors before you seek the help of essay writing services, as these can be very expensive.

Things to consider when writing

Below are some questions that are important to keep in mind when writing your personal statement:

1) ***What is it I really want the reader to know about why I want to be a PA?*** For example, are there any communities or specific populations you want to work within? Are there any areas or locations you want to impact through medicine? Who do you want to serve as a PA? What are your future plans as a PA? Are there any personal experiences that led you to your *why*?
2) ***How can I show admissions that I have prepared for this?*** Did you seek out any health or medically relevant certifications? Do you have any special skills? Describe your healthcare or patient care roles and experiences, and/or your community or volunteer experiences. Did you take any additional courses beyond the required?[12]
3) ***How can I bring aspects of my personality or character into my essay?*** For example, what are your strengths? What do your patients, coworkers, or friends say about you? Are there any experiences you can write about that you feel accurately depict your character or personality?
4) ***Did I do a good job of showing the reader that I understand the role of a PA?*** Have you shadowed a PA? Do you have a PA mentor? Are you a part of any clubs or organizations that are related to the PA profession?

---

[12] If you are reading this book, then you should have definitely taken additional coursework and this is something you may want to consider adding to your PS as a strength.

What are some specific aspects of the PA profession that you find especially interesting or that resonate with you?

5) ***If you are a reapplicant to PA school, what did you do differently this cycle?*** For example, did you obtain additional patient care experience? Did you volunteer or participate in community service? Did you continue your education?

   And last but not least:

6) ***If I had issues along the way, how did I overcome them? Were any of these character-building?*** As a low GPA applicant, you ABSOLUTELY should include this in your personal statement. Do not provide excuses or sad stories about your obstacles. Instead, you want to *briefly* provide an explanation for why you struggled, and take ownership. What is most important is that you detail what you did to overcome any obstacles you faced, and how you moved forward. If you can also detail why you think your struggles make you a strong candidate, then this is an added bonus.

When it comes time to write your personal statement, you may find it helpful to have these questions handy as you brainstorm what you want to write about. These six questions can be a guide, and although you do not need to address each of the questions within the body of your personal statement, incorporating at least three of them will ensure you have the elements that typically make for a compelling personal statement. Once you have the content and theme down of your essay, any issues with grammar, punctuation, or flow can easily be corrected by the people who have agreed to read it and give feedback, or a writing service.

Just because I like to make things crystal clear, question #6 is a must have as a low GPA applicant. I want to remind you that no matter what anyone else says, there is strength in overcoming challenges. Do not miss out on the opportunity to explain why your past challenges were just a temporary setback, and provide details of how you have moved forward. If you choose not to, it may be the difference between you being offered an interview or receiving a flat out rejection.

CHAPTER 10:
HEALTHCARE AND PATIENT CARE EXPERIENCE

My first cycle applying to PA school I had ZERO healthcare and ZERO patient care experience. Don't be like me. The more hours of experience you can accrue the better.

This is yet another component of the PA application that is of high importance for us low GPA applicants. Unlike some other healthcare professions, having prior experience in a healthcare setting is essential to your application profile. In fact, there is a section on CASPA where you will be asked to list and categorize all your experiences.

As an applicant, you need to be aware that there is a difference between healthcare experience (HCE) and patient care experience (PCE).

According to CASPA, HCE is defined as: both paid and unpaid work in a health or health-related field where you are not directly responsible for a patient's care, but may still have patient interaction. PCE is described as: experiences in which you are directly responsible for a patient's care.

To put it simply, what separates the two is really your level of involvement with patients. Is one better than the other? Not necessarily, because any experience that adds value to your pre-PA journey is beneficial.

However it is important to note that typically PA programs require that applicants have direct PCE. Some may even go as far and state direct *paid* PCE which indicates that they expect you to have previous employment history of PCE. Even the ones that don't require it will list PCE as "preferred" or "recommended." With that being said, I think it is safe to say that having PCE will really help make you a more competitive applicant.

To help clarify the differences between the two even further, below are some *examples* of jobs that fall under each category. This is by no means an all-inclusive list, as there are so many jobs in the healthcare realm.

Experience Type	Job Examples
HCE	patient transporter, medical receptionist, medical biller, unit secretary, social worker, case manager, medical interpreter, health educator, patient advocate, hospital volunteer
PCE	RN, LPN, EMT, paramedic, combat medic, military corpsman, patient care tech/associate, medical assistant, certified nursing assistant (CNA), home health aide (HHA), phlebotomist, physical therapist/aide, occupational therapist/aide, rehab aide, EKG tech, emergency room tech, dental tech/hygienist, x-ray tech, surgical assistant, respiratory therapist/aide, dietician, speech language therapist/aide

As you can see from the list above, HCE jobs are typically those that require minimal interaction with patients as it pertains to their *diagnosis*, treatment, or care. As such, these job types are classified as non-clinical. If you have minimal direct contact with patients, or find yourself doing mainly clerical or administrative work, then your role should be listed on CASPA as HCE.

PCE jobs require you to be directly involved with the patient's care and treatment. With these types of jobs, you typically work in a *clinical* setting under the direction of another care provider (think doctors, nurses, PAs, nurse practitioners), and part, if not all, of your responsibilities involve clinical work.

But what if your job has components of HCE and PCE? Can you use the same job for both sections on CASPA? This is a common question I get asked and the answer is yes! For example, if you work full-time as a medical assistant, you may spend 3 days a week doing clinical work (drawing blood, taking vitals, dressing wounds), but 2 days a week processing lab samples, organizing patient records, and stocking supplies. In this case, you would list your position as a medical assistant as both HCE and PCE. However, you will need to do a little bit of math to make sure you are accounting for the hours worked in each role. Using the example above, you would list under PCE your job as a medical assistant and the hours you accrued working 3 days a week clinically. Under HCE, you would once again put down medical assistant and record the hours you accrued working 2 days a week non-clinically.

Variable Types of Experience

With the above in mind, I want to list a few jobs that I like to classify as "variable." This is because they may qualify as HCE or PCE, depending on your level of involvement with patients and your job responsibilities as defined by your workplace. Here are a few examples of variable jobs:

Athletic trainer	Clinical research coordinator	Medical scribe
Pharmacy technician	Research assistant	Scrub tech

To help you understand further, *let* me provide you with a real-life example:

My job as a Surgical PA requires that I work closely with scrub techs— also known as surgical techs or operating room (OR) techs. In fact, I depend on them to *do* my job efficiently. During a surgical procedure, the area *surrounding* the patient needs to be made into a "sterile field." Anyone who is operating in this field as well as any surgical instruments that will be used need to be sterile. It is the duty of the scrub tech to set up and maintain this sterile field, both before and during surgery. During surgery, they are responsible for handling surgical instruments, sponges, or dressings when requested to the individuals performing the surgery. These are the typical duties of a scrub tech, and as such, this would count towards HCE.

However, at the hospital where I work, while the scrub techs are indeed responsible for *everything* I listed in the above paragraph, they also have additional duties that involve direct patient care and interaction. Once the patient is wheeled into the OR, they assist with transferring the patient to the OR table, and help with any prep that may be needed such as shaving or disinfecting the area of the body that will be operated on. During surgery, they play a role by helping to retract skin and tissue, provide suction when needed, and monitor patient status. When surgery is completed, they help clean and dress the patient, and may even accompany them to the recovery room. As you can see, the scrub techs at my hospital could list their experience as PCE.

So what point am I trying to make? If you have any of the jobs that are considered variable, it may or may not count towards a PA school's PCE requirement. Your job title might be the same as others, however your responsibilities may differ depending on where you work. From the example I provided above, a scrub tech at a different hospital may not have the PCE that the scrub techs at my hospital have. PA programs are well *aware* of this fact, so while job title is important, they are also assessing how you functioned in that role. For this reason alone, it is very important that you are very descriptive in your explanation of your job role in the relevant CASPA sections AND in your personal statement.

Also keep in mind, PA programs may list some or all of these variable experiences as unacceptable for meeting the PCE requirements on their website. If you feel like your role does qualify as direct PCE, you can and should contact that program. Whether you choose to email, talk on the phone, or speak to them *directly*, your goal is to explain to them why you feel like your job meets their qualifications. If for whatever reason you cannot get an answer from them directly about whether or not they will make an exception, then I would still go ahead and categorize it as PCE on CASPA, keeping in mind that you will still need to be specific in how you describe your job function and responsibilities so they can better understand and approve it as PCE.

My Personal Experience With This

By my third and final cycle of applying to PA school, I had accrued *approximately* 3700 hours of direct patient care experience. It took me about 2.5-3 years to build up this experience. I worked full-time as medical scribe at a busy urgent care clinic and part-time as a patient care tech on the medical intensive care unit (MICU) of a hospital simultaneously. From there, I held full-time employment as a medical assistant for a few different practices and specialties such as orthopedics, OB/GYN, and oncology.

I accrued the most hours via my medical scribe job, and to be honest, it was where I *learned* the most about medicine. In addition to my scribe duties of documenting the patient encounter, I was also expected to bring patients to the exam room, take their vitals, assist with bedside procedures, draw blood for lab tests, process urine symptoms, and go over discharge instructions with them. The providers who worked there really relied on their scribes to do their job efficiently, and would often include us in discussions about a patient's diagnoses and course of treatment.

While applying, I did come across a few programs that either did not accept medical scribe experience for their PCE requirement, or considered it to be average to lower-tiered experience. Because I knew my responsibilities as a scribe went beyond that of a typical scribe who just types on a keyboard all day, I made sure to *contact* each program directly to fill them in on my duties. By doing that, I was able to get my medical scribe experience approved as PCE. In addition, I made sure to write in detail about each of my healthcare jobs on my personal statement as well as document them in the CASPA experiences section.

As a low GPA non-traditional student, the more varied experiences you have, especially in a healthcare setting, the better your overall application will be. My upward trend in academics, coupled with my extensive patient care experience, is what got programs to pay attention to my application, and subsequently led to me getting interview invites. The sooner you can start working on gaining patient care experience, the better.

Other Important Things to Know and Remember

Some, but not all, PA programs:

- ➢ Rank PCE, which means that they may consider one job as higher or preferred versus another
- ➢ Have a minimum hour requirement for PCE
- ➢ Have no minimum hour requirement for either PCE or HCE
- ➢ Will ask for verification of hours worked
- ➢ Consider HCE and PCE as one and the same, or may lump both under the heading healthcare experience
- ➢ Will allow MD or PA shadowing as HCE

Remember that:

- ➢ As a low GPA applicant, it would be in your best interest to have PCE
- ➢ The most competitive applicants have 2000+ hours of direct PCE which is equivalent to approximately 1 year of full-time work
- ➢ The experience section on CASPA is where you will list your HCE and PCE, however, you should also include other experience types here such as volunteer, leadership, teaching, research, and shadowing
- ➢ You should go into detail and specifics about each of your experiences on CASPA and in your personal statement. Do not use generic descriptions (eg. Google medical assistant and copy and paste what the description is for that job)

CHAPTER 11: LETTERS OF RECOMMENDATION

Your letters of recommendation should provide insight to your personal strengths, character, and/or accomplishments.

Your application to PA school is not complete until you have three letters of recommendation, also known as letters of reference (LOR) on file. You can actually have up to five LORs, but only three are required to submit your application.

The way this works is on your CASPA application, you will list three to five people who you anticipate will write you a letter of recommendation under the section titled "References and Evaluations." CASPA will require you to input their full name and email address. You will then need to indicate whether or not you waive your right to view the final evaluation for each person listed. I would recommend you select 'Yes' to waive your right, as programs may view this recommendation as a more accurate and honest evaluation of your candidacy for PA school[13]

Once you have completed the required information, CASPA will then send each person you listed an email address for with a link where they will be asked to create a profile as an "Evaluator."[14] This is where they will fill in information such as their title/salutation, full name, occupation, organization or workplace, and phone number. The reference will also

---

13 See Appendix F for further information regarding waivers.

14 You may want to notify your prospective evaluators that the email will come from caspainfo@caspaonline.org and that they should also check their spam and junk folders if they do not see it in their inbox.

complete a brief survey about you as an applicant and upload the letter of recommendation they wrote for you. Once they complete and submit their evaluation, you should receive an email confirmation that an evaluation has been submitted on your behalf. However, you can utilize the 'check status' tab to view the progress of all your evaluations. You can also resend evaluation requests, as well as change, delete, or add recommenders.[15]

Now that we covered the logistics of how to input evaluators on CASPA, let me break down the more important details of how to go about obtaining LORs.

Who Should Write Your LOR

My rule of thumb for all low GPA applicants is that they should absolutely have a letter of recommendation from someone in academia, ideally from a science professor. Since you are an applicant who has had academic issues, having someone with an academic background speak to your capabilities as a student will really help paint the picture to PA programs that you are a bright individual. If you are choosing a professor, of course you will want to have done well in that course, but other options are academic advisors, department heads, or teacher assistants.

In addition to an academic reference, you should plan to have a LOR from a PA. In fact, some PA programs actually require a LOR from a PA as part of their application requirements. But whether it is required or not, a LOR from a PA will go a long way in making your application profile more competitive. If you are able to obtain an LOR from more than one PA, then you are in even better shape! Think about

---

[15] You can add a maximum of five evaluators. If you want to switch out one for another, you are able to do so, but once an individual has submitted their evaluation you can no longer delete it.

it...who better to recommend you as a future PA than someone who actually works in the profession?

After you have secured the academic and PA letter of reference, you will want to identify other individuals who you feel know you well enough to write you a glowing recommendation. It is always a good idea to obtain letters from those who know you from either a professional or educational setting. However, the best LORs come from those who have observed you in your interactions with patients, and can provide insight into your personality, character, and other positive attributes.

You also want to make sure you are asking people who have known you for some time. In fact, CASPA will ask your evaluators to indicate how long they have known you, and in what capacity. A recommendation from someone who has known you for a year or longer will typically hold more weight than someone who has only known you for two months.

How to Obtain a Quality LOR

The extent of your relationship with your evaluators is equally as important. You do not just want *any* letter of recommendation. Your goal should be to obtain ***quality*** letters of recommendation. The onus is on YOU to make sure that all letters uploaded on your behalf are glowing recommendations. So how do you ensure this?

1. Make sure you are asking the right people to serve as references for you. The people you ask should be those who have known you personally for a period of at least six months.
2. Once you have identified individuals you think will serve as great references, do your best to maintain

your relationship with them, especially if these are people you do not interact with on a daily basis.

3. Supply your recommenders with documents that can better help them write you a good LOR. Items such as a brief bio, your resume, personal statement, an outline or short summary of things you think they should include in their letter are all helpful (See Appendix G for a copy of the bio I provided my recommenders with).

This final tip may be controversial and is not absolutely necessary, but I feel it is still important to mention...

4. Ask to read a draft of the LOR they plan to submit. This can help ensure that the recommendations you receive are those of substance and quality.

I want to elaborate a bit more on this last point. All too often, I hear from colleagues that they have no idea what to write in their recommendations. This is because although they may mean well, not everyone is great at putting their thoughts into words. I myself have read LORs that are lacking in detail or are very superficial. The best LORs are those that provide real-life examples or detailed explanations of why this person thinks you have what it takes to become a PA. In addition to supplying your recommenders with documents such as a brief bio, your personal statement, or resume, you can also provide them with a set of questions that can help guide them as they write their recommendations. Here are a few examples that may help them reflect upon their relationship with you:

- Are they impressed by your bedside manner or overall demeanor? If so, why?
- Have they observed your patient interactions? If so, what if anything stands out to them?

- Are there certain qualities about you they feel make you unique?
- What characteristics or personal attributes do they think you best exhibit? (honesty, friendly, detail-oriented, team-player, attentive, compassion, organized, ethical, problem-solver, patience)
- Why do they think you are a good fit for the PA profession?

In helping them answer these questions, do not hesitate to offer specific examples or any instances that may come to mind. By offering your input as they draft their letter, or asking them if they feel comfortable enough to let you read it as they work towards a finalized LOR, you can be reassured that the letter they submit on your behalf is one that presents you in the best light possible. Keep in mind they have full discretion as to what is uploaded as a final copy, and as such, you should still indicate on CASPA that you are waiving your right to view this evaluation. (See Appendix G for more information on waivers).

My Personal Experience With This

For my third and final application cycle, I chose to utilize all five evaluation slots on my CASPA application. Even though CASPA requires a minimum of three, my thought process was the more people who could speak highly of me, the better.

I carefully considered who I should ask, and why I thought they would make great references. A few weeks before the application cycle opened, I asked each person if they would be willing to write me an LOR, and once they agreed, I sent them an email specifying why I thought they could provide an excellent reference for me. I also attached a brief bio about my upbringing, background, academic struggles, and future plans along with my resume (see Appendix H for a copy of the brief bio I provided each of them with).

It is my opinion that your evaluators can only speak to your strengths within the environment they have observed you in, however, if you provide them with additional information about yourself, this typically will help them write a more well-rounded and detailed LOR. For example, my evaluators knew me as the "Samora in the here and now," and were shocked to learn that I had failed out of college at one point in my life. By sharing this information with them, a few of them chose to write about how they thought I was a smart and dedicated individual who they felt would make an excellent future PA based on their experiences with me, in spite of my past challenges.

To help you further understand who should serve as a reference for you, I have included below some detailed information about each of the individuals who submitted an LOR on my behalf as well as why I specifically chose them:

Neurobiology professor:
I took this course during my post-bacc and received an A+. However, I specifically reached out to this professor because I was an active student in her class. I always participated in class discussions and student activities and showed interest in the course topic. In addition to this, I often met with her after class or during office hours whenever I needed help, and also shared with her my plans of becoming a PA as well as the reason why I was doing a post-bacc. I should also mention, this professor was a Chinese native and she had difficulty with writing in English. As such, she welcomed my assistance in helping her draft an LOR for me.

Chief Regional Medical Doctor (MD):

I worked closely with this doctor over the course of two years as a medical scribe. He was aware that I was an aspiring PA, and as such, he would involve me in the decision-making process for each patient he treated and allowed me to assist him with complicated procedures. He also advocated that I be promoted to chief medical scribe within six months of me being hired, and specifically requested that I be his scribe each time he worked at my clinic site because of my work ethic.

Physician Assistant (x 3):

I worked closely with each of these PAs for approximately 3.5 years and served as either their medical scribe or medical assistant. All three of them had been PAs for several years and had varied background experiences. Each of them expressed to me that they believed I had what it took to get through PA school and become an excellent PA, based on their experiences with me and their knowledge of the profession. Since I worked with each of them on many occasions and assisted in treating a broad range of patients, I knew a LOR from them would speak to my clinical skills, medical knowledge, bedside manner, and team-oriented spirit.

By communicating clearly with each of the individuals listed above why I wanted them to serve as a reference for me, as well as providing them with additional information, such as my background and personal statement, I was able to secure quality LORs. In fact, one PA program even let me know my recommendations were a huge factor in why they decided to offer me an interview.

Once your letters of recommendations are done, be sure to thank your letter writers! A genuine email or small token of appreciation shows them that you are considerate of the time and effort they put in to complete your evaluation. Expressing your gratitude will also make them more willing to serve as a reference for you in a subsequent cycle should you need to reapply.

An additional note about that. One question I get asked often is if you have to reapply to PA school, do you need to get all new recommendations? The answer is NO! You can reach out to the same individuals and they can absolutely use the same LOR or variation of it, especially if it was a good one. You would still need to list them as on CASPA so that they will receive an updated link to complete their profile as an "Evaluator."

If there is a chance you have to reapply, I always recommend that you stay in contact with those you have asked to serve as references for you and keep them updated on your progress. For example, when I did not get into PA school on my second attempt, I sent an email to each person and let them know that I would be reaching out again the following cycle. During the interim, I periodically checked in with them via email or met with them in person to catch up. When it came time to reapply, I informed them of any new changes or experiences that they should be aware of (new jobs, courses taken, etc.) Just remember, staying in contact will make it far easier for you to request a LOR from them, and less awkward.

Another tip I like to provide applicants with is that you should provide each person you need the recommendation from with plenty of time to complete your evaluation. I reached out to each person several weeks before the application cycle opened so that they could at least get a head start on writing my LOR. I also provided each person with a timeline of when I planned to submit my applications so that they were aware of when they should have their evaluations completed. As it grew closer to the dates I wanted to submit, I checked in with them periodically.

Remember, you cannot submit your application until you have at least three evaluations submitted to CASPA. If you are planning on having more than three, you can always submit your application once you have three completed evaluations, but plan to check in with the remaining individuals as soon as possible so there is not a huge gap between your application submission and their completed evaluation. It is in your best interest that PA programs evaluate all your application materials at once, and if you have one or two recommendations in progress, a program may choose to wait until they are completed before reviewing your application.

One final point, if for whatever reason you do not hear back from someone who agreed to write you a LOR after several attempts of checking in, you may want to consider deleting them from your list of evaluators. CASPA allows you to make changes to any person whose evaluation is listed as incomplete. You can choose to delete them entirely or replace them with a new evaluator as long as you have not reached the max of five. Do not let a delayed recommendation be the reason why you do not submit your PA school application in a timely fashion.

CHAPTER 12:
STANDARDIZED TESTING

As if applying to PA school wasn't already demanding, you may also have to take an exam as part of the application process.

PA schools utilize standardized testing as another data point that can help them select qualified applicants. Although I know exams can be an added source of anxiety or stress, this element of the application may actually work in your favor.

Back when I was applying to PA school, you did not need to worry about taking a standardized test, as the majority of programs had no such requirement. For the few that did, the Graduate Record Examination (GRE) was the one most commonly required for admission. Since then, two others have joined the realm of standardized tests for PA school: the PA-CAT and CASPER exam. But before I go into details about each, I want to point out a few things that low GPA applicants need to consider with standardized tests.

To Take or Not To Take the Test?

Like most other components of the PA school application process, the requirements for standardized testing will vary from program to program. There are some which have no testing requirement whatsoever, while others may prefer one exam over another, or more than one of the three exams. What is even more frustrating for applicants are the programs which make testing optional or better yet, "highly suggest" applicants take the test.

Then comes the issue of exam scores. Some programs are upfront about what numbers they are looking for, while others are pretty vague. All of this is confusing because it leaves the applicant guessing about the competitiveness of their score, and whether or not they should consider an exam retake.

This leads to a question that I am frequently asked by pre-PAs: Should you only apply to programs that do not have a standardized test requirement? Although each situation is unique, my typical response is "No," especially for those with academic issues. As a low GPA applicant, it is in your best interest to take advantage of any opportunity that will allow you to add positive elements to your application. If you happen to score well on one or more of these exams, this can potentially help offset your low GPA. On the other hand, if you happen to not perform well, programs may see this as another negative aspect of your application.

By solely applying to programs that do not have a mandatory requirement for standardized tests, you are essentially narrowing the pool of schools you can apply to. As a low GPA applicant, you are already limited in choices, so why make it even harder on yourself? However, if you keep your options open, and prepare for any exams that may be required, you will have a broader list of schools to choose from. The more programs you can apply to, the better your chances of getting an acceptance. So take the test(s)!

The Three Most Common Tests for PA School Admissions

<u>Graduate Record Examination (GRE)</u>: This test is owned and administered by the Educational Testing Service (ETS), and is an exam that is required of most applicants seeking graduate school admission within the United States. The GRE assesses knowledge of college-level English and mathematics. There are approximately 100 questions on this exam, spread out over six sections, which fall under the categories of:

- Quantitative reasoning

- ➢ Verbal reasoning
- ➢ Analytical writing

Allotted Time: 3 hours 45 minutes

Test Fee: $205

The Physician Assistant College Admission Test (PA-CAT): This test is owned by Exam Master, but what is unique about this test is that it was designed specifically for PA school admissions. In fact, PA educators assisted with the creation of this test, with the idea that it can help PA programs conduct a more holistic review of prospective candidates.[16] The test consists of 240 multiple-choice questions which cover nine subject areas:

- ➢ Anatomy
- ➢ Physiology
- ➢ General Biology
- ➢ Biochemistry
- ➢ General and Organic Chemistry
- ➢ Microbiology
- ➢ Behavioral Sciences
- ➢ Genetics
- ➢ Statistics

While this may seem like a lot, be aware that the majority of prerequisite courses required by PA school admissions are based on ALL of these subjects.

---

[16] As per the PA-CAT website: *The PA-CAT has been developed specifically for use by PA educators and their admissions departments as part of a holistic admissions process.*

Allotted Time: 4.5 hours

Test Fee: $228

Computer-Based Assessment for Sampling Personal Characteristics (CASPER): This test is owned and distributed by Altus Assessments, and differs from the other two exams as it is classified as an open-response situational judgment test (SJT). What this means is that CASPER is not another multiple-choice exam that tests your knowledge of various subject matters. Instead, the exam consists of twelve sections: eight video-based and four word-based prompts, followed by three questions. Each section is designed to assess the following personal and professional attributes:[17]

- Collaboration
- Communication
- Empathy
- Equity
- Ethics
- Motivation
- Problem solving
- Professionalism
- Resilience
- Self-awareness

Allotted Time: 90 minutes

Test Fee: $40

[17] Attributes are as listed on the CASPER test website: takealtus.com

You may be wondering what score you should aim for with each of these tests. This is not an easy thing to answer because each exam has their own scoring system. Technically, there is no "passing score" for any of three exams listed above, however scoring at or above the 50th percentile is typically considered to be competitive. You can find more information about how these exams are scored on their respective test websites in Appendix H.

It is also important to note that these exams and scores will have a different impact on your overall application depending on the program you apply to. When in doubt, it is always best to check directly with the programs.

Key Points to Remember

In Chapter 8 of this book, I detailed how to identify PA programs that will give your application a fair chance, in spite of a low GPA. Using the advice in that chapter will help you create your ideal PA school list. What I don't want to happen, is for you to cross off any schools on that list that may require you to take a test. Recognize that this is an opportunity to enhance your application, and use that along with all the other advice in this book. If your goal is to prove to programs why you deserve a seat, then go above and beyond what is required.

There are plenty of test prep materials and resources available for each of these standardized tests that you can find on their respective exam websites, on YouTube, or are shared in pre-PA Facebook groups or forums. Take the time to prepare adequately so that you can approach these exams with confidence. Your performance on the standardized tests can be the one thing that sets your application apart and encourages programs to give you a chance.

My Personal Experience With This

When I was applying to PA school, the GRE was the only standardized test I had to consider as the other two did not exist yet. In fact, I first heard of the PA-CAT and CASPER when I was in my final semester of PA school.

I will be honest and admit that I had to take the GRE four times before I received a satisfactory score. The first attempt was a few months before I applied to PA school for the second time. I did not take the test as seriously as I should have and barely studied for it. Based on the limited research I conducted prior to my exam date, the content of the GRE was based on courses I had taken in undergrad, and was not supposed to be a hard exam. I was a full-time post-bacc student and held a full-time job, so my time was very limited. Since I considered myself to have an extensive vocabulary and superb writing skills, I did even less test prep for those sections. Needless to say, I bombed the quantitative section and had a very low percentile ranking. But what was even more surprising to me was that my verbal reasoning and writing score was just average. It was clear to me that preparation was needed if I was ever going to do well. So I chose not to forward the scores from my first attempt and instead planned to retake the exam for a higher score.

Unfortunately, I let my anxiety get the best of me the second time I took the test and ran out of time. I won't even mention what my scores were, but just know I might as well have taken the exam with my eyes closed. On my third retake, I was better prepared and scored significantly higher. My verbal and writing score were in the 75th percentile, but my quantitative score was just below the 50th.[18] As such, I decided to take the test for a fourth time right before my third

---

18 Typically, GRE scores at or above the 50th percentile in each section are considered competitive.

and final cycle of applying to PA school. My scores were in the 75th percentile for every section, and I was happy to have finally met my goal.

My GRE score definitely played a role in my success as a PA school applicant. How do I know this? Well, the feedback received from a few programs after I was rejected during my second cycle applying was that I should retake the GRE and aim to get a higher score in each section. I hated the fact that I had to take this exam so many times, but I appreciated the fact this was another way to prove to PA programs that I was committed. In the end, it worked to my benefit. Of course, my GRE score was not the only thing that helped me gain acceptance, but it certainly helped! And my previously low scores on the first and second attempt did not impact me at all, since I was able to report only my highest score as part of my application.

Applying to PA school can be an arduous process with many steps. However, each step is necessary to bring you that much closer to your goal. Do not let anything stand in your way!

Part 4:

Tying It All Together

CHAPTER 13:
FORMULATING YOUR PLAN

Creating a strategic plan with actionable steps can help you feel motivated as you work towards your goal.

I remember how hopeless I felt after I was rejected from every program I applied to my first CASPA cycle. I contemplated if I should continue to pursue my goal of becoming a physician assistant or if I should follow the advice of my pre-health advisor and pick an entirely new career. Looking back now, I am so glad that I decided to take a leap of faith and do everything in my power to make myself a more appealing candidate for PA school.

The detailed chapters of this book should help you have a better understanding of the steps you need to take so that you can also find success getting into PA school with a low GPA. However, it is imperative that you use this information to help you formulate a plan to apply. The plan does not have to be super detailed, but it should be realistic and specific to your situation. I had a plan each time I applied to PA school and adjusted it as needed. This was key to helping me stay organized and motivated throughout my arduous journey.

Where to Begin with Your Plan

Reading and rereading this book is a great place to start! Highlight or bookmark pages that are relevant to where you are in the application process.

From there, I would advise you to take a close look at your transcripts and review the courses you have already taken. Ask yourself the following questions:

- Have you completed all the prerequisite courses for PA school?[19] If so, what grades did you receive? Are they at least a C? Did you get a B or higher in the majority of the prerequisite courses?
- Do you need to retake any courses for a higher grade?
- Should you register for additional science courses? If so, where will you matriculate (online versus in-person, community college versus university)?

Once you have decided on the above, come up with a rough timeline of when you would like to apply, based on when you anticipate completing some or all of the courses.

You can also start to create your ideal PA school list.[20] Research programs you are interested in, and attend events such as open houses and school fairs. The PAEA has a virtual fair at least twice a year where applicants can chat with PA program admissions personnel.[21] Events such as these are especially beneficial if you have questions that cannot be found on the program websites. You can always contact programs directly via phone or email if you need any additional information, but be sure you meet the requirements for every school you add to your list. You may need to revisit this list if you are creating it ahead of the cycle you plan to apply, or if you find yourself needing to reapply. Keep in mind that PA programs may change their requirements from cycle to cycle, so you will need to verify that you still meet the admissions requirements.

Lastly, you want to make sure you budget accordingly. Applying to PA school can be an expensive process when you

---

19 Review Chapter 1 for information regarding the prerequisite courses for admission to PA school.

20 See Chapter 8, section titled How to Craft Your PA School List.

21 Information about the virtual fair can be found on the Physician Assistant Education Association (PAEA) website: paeaonline.org

factor in costs such as standardized testing, application fees, supplemental application fees, interview travel and accommodations, etc. Once you decide to apply to PA school, you should begin saving. If possible, put away a little bit of money each paycheck. Remember, you are investing in your future!

Additional Tips When It's Time To Apply

Let's fast forward to the future. You are super confident that you have a good shot of getting into PA school because you read this book and worked hard to make yourself a competitive applicant. You are now ready to apply and want to make sure you do everything right.

Here are some additional tips to help you when it comes time to apply to PA schools:

- ➢ Apply early. You have a better chance of getting an interview offer earlier in the application cycle when programs have not yet filled all their seats
- ➢ Be aware of program deadlines so your applications can be submitted on time
- ➢ Provide detailed descriptions of each of your experiences on CASPA, especially in regard to your direct PCE
- ➢ Be aware that experiences such as leadership, volunteering, extracurriculars, awards, certifications, teaching, and research are all valuable and can help your application stand out among the rest
- ➢ Be sure to check your spam folder. Sometimes emails from programs end up in the spam or junk mail and you don't want to miss any important email from them, such as an interview invitation

I want to end this chapter with one of my favorite quotes and reminder to myself whenever I set a new goal or challenge:

"There are dreamers and there are planners;
the planners make their dreams come true."
-Edwin Louis Cole-

Chapter 14:
Final Thoughts

I can sum up my PA journey with the saying:

"Nothing worth having in life comes easy."

When I was academically dismissed from college, I thought my whole world was over. I had been a good student for most of my life up until that point, and never really had any academic issues. I thought about all the people who looked up to me and how disappointed they would be. I did not know how to tell them that I ruined my future. In fact, I was so embarrassed and so ashamed of my failures that I continued to pretend that I was in school long after I stopped attending. I had no plan in place, no idea what the future held for me, and was not ready to face my harsh reality.

Perhaps that was where you were before you found this book; lost, confused, and uncertain about your future. Maybe you were told that becoming a PA would be nearly impossible because of your mistakes. I was there too once, and was told the exact same things by so many people. I almost believed them too...

I am often asked what kept me going, and the honest answer is the little voice inside of me. Even at my lowest point in life, I heard it talking to me, reminding me of the dreams I had for my future, and nagging me to move forward. I wanted to pursue medicine, and deep down I knew I had to at least try or risk living the rest of my life with regret. If I failed, at least I would know that it wasn't due to lack of effort.

What I want you to take away from this book is that you can bounce back from your failures. But this first starts with honest self-reflection. Ask yourself, are you committed to doing the hard work? Can you handle it along with all the other things on your plate right now? Don't be afraid if the answer is no. The reality is, the journey to redemption is not an easy one and if it doesn't make sense for where you are in life currently, then that is okay. You have to do what works for you, but don't let anyone influence your decision. You and you alone know what you are and are not capable of accomplishing.

If you do choose to move forward, be prepared for more obstacles. I will not lie and tell you that it will be easy from here on out, because it won't. Even after I had a solid plan in place, I still faced disappointments and struggled to stay motivated. I hated being an older student still trying to complete undergrad. I cringed each time I had to explain to a family member or friend why I was still in school. I hated having to retake classes for a second or third time. While friends were out enjoying life and advancing their careers, there I was studying or preparing to apply to yet another application cycle. And rejections...they hurt so bad. You have all this hope after you submit your applications only to be crushed later when a school informs you that you did not make their cut. You may shed tears or become angry or discouraged several times along your journey, but I urge you to keep focused and continually look for opportunities to improve your odds.

This book *will* help you strengthen your application so that you can compete with the hundreds of other students who apply to PA school each year. But the strength to move forward has to come from within you. You will need to be patient and give yourself grace. Develop tunnel vision, follow your plan, and remind yourself as often as you need to of why you started.

I wove my story throughout this book because I have walked in your shoes and have made it to the other side. How I got here is what this book is all about, and I want you to know that you can make it here too. I have met so many students with similar stories to mine, and have helped countless others gain acceptance to PA school. All you need is one "yes," one school to acknowledge all the effort you put in and extend you the opportunity to change your life forever.

Being a physician assistant is such an amazing career with so many opportunities. You can do this. Your future self and your patients will be grateful you did not give up.

Part 5:

Additional Resources

FAQ

1. What should I major in during undergrad?

PA programs do not require applicants to have a specific major, so you are free to major in anything. However, most applicants find it easier to complete the required prerequisite courses if they major in the sciences (eg. biology, chemistry, or related).

2. Will it look bad if I switch majors during undergrad?

No, this will not count against you. You are free to major in any subject and switch as you see fit.

3. Should I address my low GPA in my personal statement?

Absolutely! Your personal statement is your opportunity to tell your story and include an explanation as to why your GPA is low in your own words. However, be brief in your explanation of why you struggled and focus more on detailing the things you did to improve your GPA.

4. Should I address my low GPA during interviews?

Yes, if it is relevant to the question you are asked. Do not feel like you have to offer this information willingly, especially if you have briefly explained your GPA issues in your personal statement (see Question #3). Also keep in mind, PA programs have reviewed your CASPA which shows your academic history.

If an interviewer asks about your GPA, try not to get nervous about it or start to think negative thoughts. All they are looking for is for you to reassure them that you are capable of succeeding as a PA student. Remember, they offered you an interview so that they can get to know you better.

5. **Do I need to join the AAPA and/or my state chapter of physician assistants?**

Joining any PA organization can help show program admissions you are committed to the profession. CASPA has a place for professional memberships, so this is also something you can include to help your application stand out further. Many organizations offer free or discounted memberships for pre-PAs as well as other resources that may be helpful to you on your journey.

6. **When can I apply to PA schools?**

You can apply to PA school once you have met the requirements for the schools on your list and completed your CASPA.

7. **Should I do post-bacc courses at a four-year university or community college?**

Do whatever works best for you. You will hear sometimes that you should not take classes at a community college because PA programs frown upon this. While this may be true for some schools, do what is best for you. All that is important is that you achieve high grades wherever you decide to take courses. Classes at community college tend to be cheaper than those taken at the university level. However, most upper-level courses are only offered at the university level.

8. **Why should I take more than one class at a time during a post-bacc?**

It is very easy for someone to take one class and get an A in it, but can you take 2+ science courses at a time and still get As? This is what PA programs will be assessing, especially because you have had academic issues in the past. The PA school curriculum is very rigorous, so they want to make sure you have what it takes to succeed. Taking multiple courses and doing well in all of them will help PA programs see the kind of student you are presently.

9. Should I do an MPH?

If you need to improve your science GPA, then an MPH is **not** the right degree for you. You should focus on taking classes that are science and/or medical related as this can help you offset your low GPA.

10. What if I have retaken a course multiple times?

This will be a red flag to programs, so before you attempt the course again, try to address why you are struggling.

If there is another course you can take in its place that is a similar subject, then take this course instead, as some PA programs allow for substitution. For example, some programs will allow biochemistry and organic chemistry to replace general chemistry.

11. Which job is best for meeting the direct patient care experience requirement/hours?

There are several jobs that qualify as direct patient care (see Chapter 10). As such, one cannot be singled out as the "best." What's important is that you do your best to seek employment at a place that will allow you to have interactions with patients daily. As an added tip, try to work for a place that employs PAs so that you have easy access to PAs you can shadow and/or ask for letters of recommendation.

12. Can I get into PA school with a misdemeanor or felony?

PA programs require a background check prior to admission. Depending on what your charges are, you may face difficulty with getting in, but it would be best to disclose these to your programs of interest beforehand to make sure you are eligible to apply.

You should also be aware that you may face obstacles with getting clinical rotations and medical licensure as both require background checks as well and have their own criteria as to what is and is not acceptable.

13. How do I know if I meet the criteria for a PA program?

Do your research! Start with the program website, attend informational sessions, and reach out to current or past students. You can also contact programs directly via phone or email.

14. How many hours of HCE or direct PCE should I have?

Some programs have their own set of requirements for HCE and/or PCE, so check their program website for more information. However, having at least 1000 hours of PCE should put you within the competitive range.

15. Can I switch out one letter of recommendation for another?

You can make changes to your evaluators so long as they have not completed and submitted their evaluation on CASPA.

16. Should I have more than three letters of recommendation (LOR)?

CASPA allows up to five LORs, but you only need to have three uploaded to your application before you can submit. The more people you can get to speak (or write) highly of you, the better it is for you, so don't turn away any potential letter writers.

17. Do I need an LOR from a PA?

Some programs have a requirement that one of your LORs has to be from a PA. Regardless, it is a good idea to try to get an LOR from a PA who knows you well.

APPENDIX A: COMMON PA SPECIALTIES

PAs work in a variety of settings and work within a broad range of specialities just like physicians.

Primary Care

- Family Medicine
- Pediatrics
- Geriatrics
- General Internal Medicine

Internal Medicine Subspecialties

- Cardiology
- Critical Care
- Endocrinology
- Gastroenterology
- Infectious Disease
- Neurology
- Hematology and Oncology
- Nephrology
- Pulmonology
- Rheumatology

Emergency Medicine

Urgent Care

Obstetrics and Gynecology

Surgical Subspecialties

- General surgery
- Cardiovascular/cardiothoracic surgery
- Orthopedic surgery
- Bariatric surgery
- Plastic surgery
- Colorectal surgery
- Neurosurgery
- Transplant surgery
- Trauma surgery
- Vascular surgery
- Head and neck surgery
- Urology

Other Physician Assistant Specialties

- Otolaryngology (ENT)
- Allergy and Immunology
- Dermatology
- Hospice and Palliative Care
- Nuclear Medicine
- Addiction Medicine
- Pain Management

- Hospital Medicine
- Psychiatry
- Occupational Health
- Ophthalmology
- Physical Medicine and Rehabilitation
- Public Health
- Radiation Oncology
- Preventative Medicine

Appendix B:
CASPA Grade Breakdown Snapshot

CASPA
Oregon Health & Science University
GPA Information

Charles, Samora
APPLICANT ID: 424XXXXX

GPAs by Subject

Subject	Hours	Quality Points	GPA
Behavioral Sciences	9.00	27.0	3.00
BCP Totals	137.00	288.1	2.10
Biology/Zoology	85.00	228.1	2.68
English	12.00	39.9	3.32
Inorganic Chemistry	26.00	23.3	0.90
Mathematics	35.00	40.6	1.16
Organic Chemistry	10.00	9.9	0.99
Other Non-Science	32.00	101.9	3.18
Other Sciences	18.00	63.9	3.55
Physics	12.00	16.0	1.33
Biochemistry	4.00	10.8	2.70

GPAs by Year

Year	Hours	Quality Points	GPA
Freshman	29.00	73.8	2.54
Sophomore	113.00	180.9	1.60
Junior	23.00	51.0	2.22
Senior	34.00	99.4	2.92
Baccalaureate	199.00	405.1	2.04
Post-Baccalaureate	35.00	126.6	3.62
Cumulative Undergraduate	234.00	531.7	2.27
Graduate	9.00	29.7	3.30
Overall	243.00	561.4	2.31
Freshman Science	8.00	22.8	2.85
Sophomore Science	57.00	46.5	0.82
Junior Science	19.00	51.0	2.68
Senior Science	30.00	87.4	2.91
Baccalaureate Science	114.00	207.7	1.82
Post-Baccalaureate Science	32.00	114.6	3.58
Cumulative Undergraduate Science	146.00	322.3	2.21
Graduate Science	9.00	29.7	3.30
Overall Science	155.00	352.0	2.27
Freshman Non-Science	21.00	51.0	2.43
Sophomore Non-Science	56.00	134.4	2.40
Junior Non-Science	4.00	0.0	0.00
Senior Non-Science	4.00	12.0	3.00
Baccalaureate Non-Science	85.00	197.4	2.32
Post-Baccalaureate Non-Science	3.00	12.0	4.00
Cumulative Undergraduate Non-Science	88.00	209.4	2.38
Graduate Non-Science	0.00	0.0	0.00
Overall Non-Science	88.00	209.4	2.38

Application Page 11

Printed on 2015-10-30 11:40AM

APPENDIX C:
MY POST-BACC COURSE LIST

CASPA
Trine University (Developing Program)
Colleges Attended & Coursework

Charles, Samora
APPLICANT ID: 424XXXXX

LONG ISLAND UNIVERSITY - C.W. POST CAMPUS : Completed

Academic Status: Freshman Year: 2003 Term: Semester/Fall								
BIO 1M	Mech of Life Processes Lect/Lab	Biology	B-	B-		4.0		Not Applicable
COLL 101	Freshman Seminar	Orientation	P	None		1.0		Not Applicable
ENG 1	Composition- Writing Across Curriculum	Composition	A-	A-		3.0		Not Applicable
MTH 3	Prep Mth for Sci Majors	Mathematics	D	D		4.0		Repeated

LONG ISLAND UNIVERSITY - C.W. POST CAMPUS : Completed

Academic Status: Freshman Year: 2004 Term: Semester/Spring								
BIO 1S	Strategies of Life-Lect & Lab	Biology	B	B		4.0		Not Applicable
EEE 1	Coop Ed Pre-placement Seminar	Special Topics	P	None		0.0		Not Applicable
ENG 2	Comp: Argument/Analy	Composition	C+	C+		3.0		Not Applicable
HIS 4	Amer Civ since 1877	History	A-	A-		3.0		Not Applicable
MTH 3	Prep Mth for Sci Majors	Mathematics	D	D		4.0		Repeated
MUS 97N	Music Critique	Music	A	A		1.0		Not Applicable
POL 1	Intro Pol Science 1	Political Science	B+	B+		3.0		Not Applicable

LONG ISLAND UNIVERSITY - C.W. POST CAMPUS : Completed

Academic Status: Freshman Year: 2004 Term: Semester/Summer 1								
EEE 2	Co-Op Work Experience	Health Education	P	None		0.0		Not Applicable

LONG ISLAND UNIVERSITY - C.W. POST CAMPUS : Completed

Academic Status: Sophomore Year: 2004 Term: Semester/Fall								
BIO 121	Intro to Human Genetics	Genetics	B	B		3.0		Not Applicable
CHM 3	Principles of Chemistry	Chemistry	D	D		4.0		Not Applicable
MTH 3	Prep Mth for Sci Majors	Mathematics	C-	C-		4.0		Repeated
PHL 13	Human Values	Philosophy	C	C		3.0		Not Applicable
POL 2	Intro Pol Science 2	Political Science	B+	B+		3.0		Not Applicable

SUNY - STONY BROOK : Completed

Academic Status: Sophomore Year: 2005 Term: Semester/Spring								
BIO 203	Cellular and Organ Physiology	Physiology	F	F		4.0		Repeated
CHE 130	Problem Solving in General Chemistry	Chemistry	U	None		0.0		Not Applicable
CHE 131	General Chemistry 1	Chemistry	NC	None		4.0		Repeated
HIS 396	Topics in US History	History	C+	C+		3.0		Not Applicable

Application Page 13

Printed on 2016-03-18 03:23PM

CASPA
Trine University (Developing Program)
Colleges Attended & Coursework

Charles, Samora
APPLICANT ID: 424XXXXX

SUNY - STONY BROOK : Completed

Academic Status: Sophomore Year: 2005 Term: Semester/Spring

MAT 123	Introduction to Calculus	Calculus	NC	None		3.0		Repeated

SUNY - STONY BROOK : Completed

Academic Status: Sophomore Year: 2005 Term: Semester/Fall

BIO 208	Cell, Brain, Mind	Biology	D	D		3.0		Not Applicable
CHE 131	General Chemistry 1	Chemistry	C	C		4.0		Repeated
HUM 202	Film & TV: History & Theory	Film/Media	B-	B-		3.0		Not Applicable
MAT 123	Introduction to Calculus	Calculus	D+	D+		3.0		Repeated

SUNY - STONY BROOK : Completed

Academic Status: Sophomore Year: 2006 Term: Semester/Spring

BIO 320	General Genetics	Genetics	C	C		3.0		Not Applicable
CHE 132	General Chemistry 2	Chemistry	F	F		4.0		Repeated
CLT 361	Literature and Society	Literature	A	A		3.0		Not Applicable
MAT 125	Calculus A	Calculus	D	D		3.0		Repeated

SUNY - STONY BROOK : Completed

Academic Status: Sophomore Year: 2006 Term: Semester/Summer 1

CHE 133	General Chemistry Lab 1	Chemistry	C+	C+		1.0		Not Applicable
MAT 125	Calculus A	Calculus	C+	C+		3.0		Repeated

NASSAU COMMUNITY COLLEGE : Completed

Academic Status: Sophomore Year: 2006 Term: Semester/Fall

BIO 214	Microbiology	Microbiology	B+	B+		4.0		Not Applicable
CHE 152	Inorganic Chemistry2	Inorganic Chemistry	F	F		4.0		Not Applicable
ENG 301	Shkspr Comdy & Hist	English	B+	B+		3.0		Not Applicable
HIS 221	Afro-Caribbean World	History	B	B		3.0		Not Applicable

SUNY - STONY BROOK : Completed

Academic Status: Sophomore Year: 2007 Term: Semester/Spring

BIO 203	Cellular and Organ Physiology	Physiology	F	F		4.0		Repeated
BIO 334	Principles of Neurobiology	Neurobiology	F	F		3.0		Not Applicable
CHE 132	General Chemistry 2	Chemistry	F	F		4.0		Repeated

Application Page 14 Printed on 2016-03-18 03:23PM

CASPA
Trine University (Developing Program)
Colleges Attended & Coursework

Charles, Samora
APPLICANT ID: 424XXXXX

SUNY - STONY BROOK : Completed

Academic Status: Sophomore Year: 2007 Term: Semester/Spring									
CHE 134	General Chemistry Lab 2	Chemistry	D	D		1.0		Not Applicable	

SUNY - STONY BROOK : Completed

Academic Status: Sophomore Year: 2007 Term: Semester/Summer 1									
PHY 121	Physics for Life Sciences 1	Physics	F	F		3.0		Not Applicable	
PHY 123	Physics for Life Sciences Lab 1	Physics	F	F		1.0		Not Applicable	

SUNY - STONY BROOK : Completed

Academic Status: Sophomore Year: 2007 Term: Semester/Summer 2									
MAT 126	Calculus B	Calculus	F	F		3.0		Not Applicable	
PHY 122	Physics for Life Sciences 2	Physics	W	None		3.0		Not Applicable	
PHY 124	Physics for Life Sciences Lab 2	Physics	W	None		1.0		Not Applicable	

SUNY - STONY BROOK : Completed

Academic Status: Sophomore Year: 2007 Term: Semester/Fall									
AMS 110	Probability & Statistics Life Sciences	Statistics	F	F		3.0		Not Applicable	
BIO 325	Animal Development	Developmental Biology	D	D		3.0		Not Applicable	
BIO 328	Mammalian Physiology	Physiology	F	F		3.0		Not Applicable	
CHE 321	Organic Chemistry 1	Organic Chemistry	F	F		4.0		Not Applicable	

CUNY - CITY COLLEGE : Completed

Academic Status: Sophomore Year: 2011 Term: Semester/Spring									
PSY 10200	Psy in Modern World	Psychology	A	A		3.0		Not Applicable	
SPAN 12100	Intro Spanish 1	Foreign Languages	A	A		4.0		Not Applicable	
SPCH 11100	Speech Foundations	Public Speaking	B	B		3.0		Not Applicable	
WHUM 10200	World Humanities 2	Humanities	A+	A+		3.0		Not Applicable	

CUNY - CITY COLLEGE : Completed

Academic Status: Junior Year: 2011 Term: Semester/Summer 1									
BIO 20700	Biology of Organisms	Biology	A-	A-		4.0		Not Applicable	

Application Page 15

Printed on 2016-03-18 03:23PM

CASPA
Trine University (Developing Program)
Colleges Attended & Coursework

Charles, Samora
APPLICANT ID: 4240354459

CUNY - CITY COLLEGE : Completed

Academic Status: Junior Year: 2011 Term: Semester/Fall									
CHEM 10401	General Chem Lecture-Lab 2	Chemistry	C	C		4.0		Not Applicable	
MATH 20900	Elements of Calculus and Statistics	Statistics	F	F		4.0		Repeated	
PHYS 20300	General Physics 1	Physics	B	B		4.0		Not Applicable	

CUNY - CITY COLLEGE : Completed

Academic Status: Junior Year: 2012 Term: Semester/Spring									
BIO 22900	Cellular and Molecular Biology	Cellular & Molecular Biology	B+	B+		4.0		Not Applicable	
CHEM 26100	Organic Chemistry 1	Organic Chemistry	D	D		3.0		Repeated	
CHEM 26101	Organic Chem 1 Workshop	Organic Chemistry	P	None		0.0		Not Applicable	

CUNY - CITY COLLEGE : Completed

Academic Status: Senior Year: 2012 Term: Semester/Summer 1									
MATH 20900	Elements of Calculus and Statistics	Statistics	B	B		4.0		Repeated	
BIO 45405	Sensory Perception	Biology	A-	A-		3.0		Not Applicable	

CUNY - CITY COLLEGE : Completed

Academic Status: Senior Year: 2012 Term: Semester/Fall									
BIO 31804	Symbiosis	Biology	A-	A-		3.0		Not Applicable	
BIO 35500	Analy: Using Create	Biology	B+	B+		4.0		Not Applicable	
CHEM 26100	Organic Chemistry 1	Organic Chemistry	C+	C+		3.0		Repeated	
SCI 31353	Health & Wellness	Health	A-	A-		3.0		Not Applicable	

CUNY - CITY COLLEGE : Completed

Academic Status: Senior Year: 2013 Term: Semester/Spring									
BIO V1800	Graduate Immunology: Lec	Immunology	C	C		3.0		Not Applicable	
BIO 31717	Genetics of Autism	Genetics	A	A		3.0		Not Applicable	
PHYS 20400	General Physics 2	Physics	D	D		4.0		Not Applicable	

CUNY - MEDGAR EVERS COLLEGE : Completed

Academic Status: Senior Year: 2013 Term: Semester/Spring									
BIO 251	Human Anatomy and Physiology 1	Anatomy	B	B		4.0		Not Applicable	
BIOL 251	Human Anatomy and Physiology Lab 1	Anatomy	P	None		0.0		Not Applicable	

Application Page 16

Printed on 2016-03-18 03:23PM

CASPA
Trine University (Developing Program)
Colleges Attended & Coursework

Charles, Samora
APPLICANT ID: 424XXXXX

CUNY - MEDGAR EVERS COLLEGE : Completed

Academic Status: Post-Baccalaureate Year: 2013 Term: Semester/Fall

BIO 252	Human Anatomy and Physiology 2	Anatomy	A-	A-		4.0		Not Applicable	
BIOL 252	Human Anatomy and Physiology Lab 2	Anatomy	P	None		0.0		Not Applicable	
BIO 261	Microbiology & Immunology	Microbiology	B+	B+		4.0		Not Applicable	
BIOL 261	Microbiology & Immunology Lab	Microbiology	P	None		0.0		Not Applicable	
BIO 323	Pathophysiology	Pathophysiology	B+	B+		3.0		Not Applicable	

CUNY - MEDGAR EVERS COLLEGE : Completed

Academic Status: Post-Baccalaureate Year: 2014 Term: Semester/Spring

BIO 351	Endocrinology	Endocrinology	A-	A-		4.0		Not Applicable	
BIO 370	Environmental Science	Environmental Science	A-	A-		3.0		Not Applicable	
BIOL 351	Endocrinology Lab	Endocrinology	P	None		0.0		Not Applicable	
HSC 210	Nutrition	Nutrition	A	A		3.0		Not Applicable	
PSYC 229	Life-span Development Psychology	Life Span Development	A+	A+		3.0		Not Applicable	

CUNY - MEDGAR EVERS COLLEGE : Completed

Academic Status: Post-Baccalaureate Year: 2014 Term: Semester/Fall

BIO 365	Human Genome	Biology	A	A		3.0		Not Applicable	
BIO 463	Molecular Neurobiology	Neurobiology	A+	A+		4.0	3.0	Not Applicable	
BIOL 463	Molecular Neurobiology Lab	Neurobiology	P	None	A+	0.0	1.0	Not Applicable	
CHM 341	Biochemistry	Biochemistry	B-	B-		4.0		Not Applicable	
CHML 341	Biochemistry Lab	Biochemistry	P	None	B-	0.0		Not Applicable	

SUNY HEALTH SCIENCE CENTER - BROOKLYN : Completed

Academic Status: Graduate Year: 2014 Term: Semester/Fall

EPID 5200	Principles of Epidemiology	Epidemiology	B+	B+		3.0		Not Applicable	

SUNY HEALTH SCIENCE CENTER - BROOKLYN : Completed

Academic Status: Graduate Year: 2015 Term: Semester/Spring

EOHS 5200	Issues in Environmental Health	Public Health	B+	B+		3.0		Not Applicable	
HPMG 5206	Intro to Health Policy and Management	Public Health	B+	B+		3.0		Not Applicable	

Application Page 17

Printed on 2016-03-18 03:23PM

CASPA
Trine University (Developing Program)
Colleges Attended & Coursework

Charles, Samora
APPLICANT ID: 424XXXXX

SUNY HEALTH SCIENCE CENTER - BROOKLYN: Planned/In Progress

Academic Status: Graduate Year: 2015 Term: Semester/Fall									
BIO 5200	Principles of Biostatistics	Biostatistics				0.0		Not Applicable	
CHSC 5200	Health Behavior and Risk Reduction	Public Health				0.0		Not Applicable	

Application Page 18

Printed on 2016-03-18 03:23PM

Appendix D:
PA Program Examples

The list below provides only a *few* examples of PA programs for each category heading. But you should know there are definitely more programs that could be added to each category. However, as PA programs may change their admissions requirements from cycle to cycle, it would be more prudent for you to conduct your own research. My goal in providing you with these examples is to show you the key words/phrases and search techniques that can help you identify additional programs on your own when it comes time for you to apply.

Disclaimer: The information listed for each program below is accurate as of November 2021 and is only a snapshot of the complete admissions requirement for each program. You will need to do your own due diligence to read the admissions requirement in their entirety.

Most Recent Credit Hours

Below are three examples of programs that recognize the most recent credit hours in their GPA requirements for admissions.

Western Michigan University PA Program located in Kalamazoo, MI is pretty straightforward as it pertains to their admissions requirement. Here is a snapshot from their website:

- ➢ An undergraduate degree, earned prior to the fall start date of the WMU PA program curriculum.
- ➢ A minimum of 1,000 hours of health care experience, which must include direct patient contact. Shadowing experiences do not count toward this requirement.

Volunteer hours may be considered at half of the total amount if direct patient care is evident.

- A minimum GPA of 3.0 in the most recent 60 credit hours.
- Six required prerequisite courses, completed prior to Dec. 31, with a grade of C or above.

As you can see from the bolded section, their GPA requirement is that you have at least a 3.0 in the last 60 credits of courses taken.

Harding University PA Program located in Searcy, Arkansas is another program that will consider most recent credit hours, however, this is not as evident at first glance. The admissions requirement posted on their website states the following:
*All Applicants must have a **minimum Cumulative Undergraduate GPA of 3.00 on a 4.00 scale** as computed by CASPA.*

However, if you were to read further, you would see the following:

*The Program may consider applications with a Cumulative Undergraduate GPA below the required 3.0 if it is clear, based on the Program review of the application, that there is strong evidence that the applicant has demonstrated current academic success. **This is based on the GPA for the last 40 hours of academic work, the academic load being carried and the level of coursework taken.** All such reviews are performed at the sole discretion of the Program.*

Translation? This program may consider your application even if you do not have a 3.0 **IF** you have performed exceptionally well in your last 40 credits. There is one caveat though; although they will make an exception for the

cumulative GPA requirement, they do expect your prerequisite GPA to be at or above a 3.0. From their website:
All applicants must have a ***required prerequisite GPA of a 3.00*** *or higher on a 4.00 scale as computed by the Program. There are no exceptions made on this minimum prerequisite GPA.*

UNC School of Medicine in Chapel Hill, NC is another great example. Their program will consider applicants with a cumulative undergraduate GPA less than 3.0, as long as the GPA for the most recent 60 credits is at least a 3.0. However, they do have a prerequisite GPA requirement as seen from the snapshot below:
Applicants must meet the following GPA thresholds (no exceptions):

Minimum cumulative GPA (all courses taken at all levels) ***or last 60 credit hours > 3.0***

Minimum cumulative prerequisite GPA > 3.2

3.0 in Completed Bachelor's Degree

Towson University PA Program located in Towson, MD is a great example in this category. It also serves as an example of why I always advise applicants to go beyond the general admissions section of program websites when conducting their research.

This may not be obvious when you first visit their PA program website, however, complete information about their admissions process can be found in their 'Physician Assistant Program Application and Admissions Information Booklet.' This booklet can be accessed via a link on the Admissions Requirements section of their website. There you will find the following listed for GPA requirement:

"minimum 3.0 GPA for completed bachelor's degree or any graduate degree; minimum science GPA of 3.0".

This program was one of the ones on my list back when I was an applicant, but before I applied, I contacted the program to make sure I met their GPA standards. It took me over four years to complete my undergraduate education and I attended four different colleges before finally completing my degree requirements. At the time I graduated with a Bachelor of Science in Biology, my cumulative GPA at this university was a 3.0. After sharing this information with Towson, they assured me that since I had a 3.0 GPA for this degree, I met their criteria for admissions. I can't reiterate enough how important it is to seek clarification from programs if you are ever unsure about their requirements!

Interestingly enough, this program would also qualify for the Most Recent Credit Hours category. Upon additional review of the Admissions Requirements section of their website, the following is listed:

*A bachelor's or master's degree from a regionally accredited college or university** with a GPA of 3.00 for full admission*

If you pay close attention, there are two asterisks (**) next to the word university, indicating that interested applicants should: **See **Exceptions to Policy** in Graduate Admissions. This last statement is a hyperlink which takes you to their Graduate Admissions Policy page, where it states the following as a condition for full admission:

Students admitted to full status must meet the basic minimum requirements of the university, plus the additional requirements of the individual program. In order to meet the basic minimum requirements for full admission to the university an applicant must have:

- Earned a baccalaureate degree from a regionally accredited college or university, with a minimum GPA of 3.00 (on a 4-point scale) in either the cumulative units of the degree **or the last 60 units of the degree, or**

- Earned a master's degree or doctorate from a regionally accredited college or university.

In cases where the above minimum standards are not met, the last 60 units may include courses taken beyond the baccalaureate degree that are 300-level or higher…

It goes on to state more information about their admission processes, but the key takeaway point I want to make is that it may take a bit of detective work on your part when you are reviewing information found on program websites. Pay attention to hyperlinks and symbols that may direct you to additional helpful information.

Replacement or Qualifying GPA

Eastern Virginia Medical School located in Norfolk VA uses the exact terms 'qualifying GPA' and 'replacement GPA' in their admissions information. Their website links to an Admissions Guidebook, which details all the necessary information for interested applicants. In this guidebook, there is a section dedicated to GPAs under 'General Admissions Requirements' and the following is stated:

Qualifying GPA- *all applicants must have one of the three qualifying GPAs described below at 3.00 or better (on a 4.0 scale as calculated by CASPA) for consideration.*

The highest of the following three possible GPAs will be scored:

1. *Actual undergraduate GPA (applicants with foreign education are considered on a case-by-case basis)*
2. *Completed U.S. graduate degree GPA or*

3. **A replacement GPA** *computed from the most recent 40 semester credit hours of U.S. coursework. Applicants without 40 credits completed in the U.S. will not qualify for a replacement GPA. This is a one-time calculation from the information listed on the CASPA application at the time we process and screen an applicant and will not be re-calculated in spite of completing additional courses.*

As you can see, they provide three different options for applicants to meet their 3.0 GPA requirement. Option 2 and Option 3 is what will probably apply to you whether you chose to continue your education as a graduate or post-bacc student. Regardless of which route chosen, if you were able to maintain a GPA of at least a 3.0, then you would meet the minimum GPA requirement for this program.

As an added note, I suppose this program also falls under the 'Most Recent Credit Hours' category based on the fact that one of their options for qualifying GPA is the last 40 credits taken. With this in mind, the term 'replacement GPA' applies to any program that allows for exceptions to their posted GPA requirements, such as prerequisite course GPA, degree GPA, or most recent credits GPA.

Admissions Appeal or Petition

Touro College in New York offers a PA program at three different campuses within the state (not to be confused with Touro University in California, which also has a PA program). The admissions information for each campus is the same.
One look at their admission requirements page may have you second guessing if you have a shot with their program. Yes indeed, they state that they have a 3.0 minimum cumulative and science GPA requirement. But don't count them out just

yet! If you look further, there is a section titled 'Admissions Appeals' and the following is stated:

Students who do not meet established grade point standards or other established admission requirements detailed above may petition the PA Admissions Committee in writing for consideration. The petition must accompany the application. It should clearly explain extenuating circumstances that have prevented the student from meeting existing grade point standards or other requirements, and describe elements of the applicant's background that would indicate the potential for success in the program. The Admissions Committee may choose to admit students who have not met established admission requirements, based on the student's petition, application, interview and other supporting documents required as part of the application process. For applicants who already hold a B.A. or B.S. degree, prerequisite courses of certain types may be waived at the discretion of the PA Program Director.

Frostburg University located in Frostburg, MD is another great example. Once again, at first glance, you may think you do not meet the criteria, as it states in bold that a 3.0 cumulative GPA is required. However, the following paragraph can also be found on the Admissions Requirements section of their program website:

As a policy, FSU Master of Medical Science in Physician Assistant Studies program does not round-up any GPA. This also applies to prospective applicant prerequisite GPAs. However, if your cumulative undergraduate total GPA is below 3.0 on a 4.0 scale, and specifically only for the cumulative overall undergraduate GPA, we are mindful that some students do poorly in their freshman year but then excel in their remaining undergraduate years. Here in the PA Program, we view this as a sign of academic and emotional maturity. If you are such a student, and only once your application has been completed and verified by CASPA, you may email Vichuda Wachs (vwachs@frostburg.edu) and request that the program reevaluate your transcripts. The program may then recalculate your overall GPA based on your Junior and Senior course grades at a 4-year regionally accredited college or university. Courses completed at a community college and courses taken alone (i.e., not with a full semester course load) will not be included in this recalculation. It is important to understand that this is done on a case-by-case basis and the program decision regarding permitting the recalculation and the results of the recalculation are final and not open to consideration for appeal. Regardless of the outcome, all applicants must still have a cumulative prerequisite grade point average of 3.0 or higher as noted above. Students requesting this exception may be asked to provide more information related to the reasons for academic performance.

Although there is no guarantee that your admissions appeal or petition for consideration will be granted, at least these programs are open to further review of applicants that do not meet their mandatory GPA requirement.

GPA 2.75 cumulative and/or science GPA < 3.0

University of Utah located in Salt Lake City, UT accepts applicants with GPAs less than a 3.0. The following is listed on their website as part of their minimum requirements for admissions:

We will review applicants whose total and science GPAs are calculated by CASPA to be at least 2.70, though we recommend a GPA above 3.0 to be a competitive applicant. A strong science GPA is preferred, and competitive applicants will tend to fall within higher GPA ranges of cumulative and science GPAs. All coursework is considered in your GPA calculation, including old coursework that has been repeated for a better grade.

Samuel Merritt University located in Oakland, CA has a slightly higher GPA requirement, but it is still less than a 3.0. A snapshot of their GPA requirements is as follows:

- Minimum cumulative GPA of 2.8 as calculated by CASPA;
- Minimum science GPA of 2.8 as calculated by CASPA;

<u>Suggested, Recommended, or Preferred GPA or No GPA listed</u>

Duke University located in Durham, NC is considered one of the top PA programs, and if you remember from Chapter 1, this is where the PA profession started. I have found that because of this, many applicants, especially those with low undergraduate GPAs, are intimidated and choose not to apply. However, this program is one that proudly states they conduct a holistic review of applicants, which is evidenced by the fact that they do not have a minimum GPA requirement. Even still, your application will definitely need to demonstrate that you have what it takes to succeed academically. The FAQ section of their website states the following:

While we do not have a minimum, GPA or GRE, if your academic performance falls significantly below our lowest range, you will need to work to improve those scores to be a competitive applicant.

Similarly, **Stanford Medicine located in Stanford, CA** has the following listed on their website as part of their minimum requirements for admissions:

While our students have strong records of academic achievement, we do not have a minimum GPA requirement, and we do not require completion of the GRE, MCAT, or PA-CAT; we will review all eligible applications regardless of prior coursework, test completion, or test scores.

If you work hard at improving your grades, and have taken a significant number of courses as part of your 'GPA Fix,' then I would strongly advise you to consider programs such as these. I know several applicants with GPAs at or below a 3.0 that have been accepted to both of these schools in particular.

Appendix E: My Personal Statement

I was introduced to the PA profession during my first shift as a hospital volunteer. It was there that I took notice of a young African American female wearing a white coat; it was her glasses that first drew my attention, as they were similar to the ones I was wearing. As I observed her from afar, an alarm suddenly began to ring, followed by a blue flashing light, and off she ran, accompanied by a swarm of white coats and scrubs.

I followed close behind, wheeling the crash cart I knew would be needed, and then stood by to take in the scene that was unfolding before me. I watched as she began the first round of chest compressions while directing the surrounding team of medical workers as to the next steps to save the patient's life. Her ID badge swayed vigorously while she skillfully performed CPR, causing my eyes to zone in on the bold red initials PA-C written below her name. I was immediately curious; what was a PA-C? Her assertiveness and leadership in this emergency situation made it clear that she was of great influence in the hierarchy of hospital personnel.

My subsequent shifts were exciting for me as I looked forward to interacting with this PA and learning all I could about her role on the medical team. Our conversations, along with my observations of her expertise, genuine care, and attentiveness for each patient left an indelible impression on me. I wanted to be the kind of health care provider *she* was, and I made the decision then to dedicate my future efforts to becoming a PA.

I began college shortly after this experience. Having been an excellent student all throughout elementary and secondary education, I had no doubt that I would continue to excel at the university level. Unfortunately, my academic record received a devastating blow during my sophomore year. This was the result of my father's choice to officially estrange me from the family following my decision to live on campus.

I was raised in a very strict and religious household, in which my interaction with people outside of the family or church was extremely limited and scrupulously monitored. I was forced to live a very sheltered and controlled lifestyle, and I felt that the move was necessary for me to become a well-rounded individual. I tried to cope with my sudden alienation, but I was deeply saddened, and I found it extremely difficult to concentrate on my courses. After several semesters of failing grades, I was informed that I was academically dismissed and could no longer attend classes at that university.

Rather than enroll at a new university, I took the time to conquer my personal obstacles while partaking in new endeavors. I participated in a service learning opportunity in Uganda, and served as a mentor with an educational-based program for young adults. I enjoyed the weeks I spent there and was reminded of how satisfying it is to help and serve others. When I returned to the U.S, I continued to immerse myself in healthcare by shadowing PAs of various specialties, and I gained valuable insight as to the daily regimen, requirements, and versatility of the PA practice. My excitement and desire to ultimately achieve this career compelled me to return to school and successfully complete my undergraduate education.

Although my past hardships may have tainted my credibility as a student, my determination and confidence in my ability to become a great PA has kept me motivated to see this goal through to the end. I have made great strides over the past five years in regards to my future as a PA. I enrolled in vocational training and earned several health-related certifications that have enabled me to work and gain experience in a variety of healthcare settings. I returned to school as a post-baccalaureate student and completed upper-level science courses in anticipation of the intense curriculum of a PA program. I recently completed graduate coursework towards a certificate program in public health, as I feel a comprehensive understanding of community health issues, especially in underserved populations, will make me a better clinician.

My work experiences are also preparing me for a career in medicine. I currently work as a medical assistant at a cancer research center where I have the opportunity to interact with patients on a more intimate level. I work alongside a team of breast oncologists, physician assistants, and nurses to help provide treatment and support to our patients and their families. I am responsible for obtaining patient vitals and medical history, and help facilitate inpatient/outpatient procedures. I am also asked to accompany patients to the infusion center for their first treatment as this process can be very overwhelming.

I previously worked as a senior medical scribe in an urgent care facility and it was my job to help provide quality patient care by assisting the attending doctor or physician assistant during examinations. My duties included interviewing patients, performing non-invasive procedures, and ensuring that patients understand the details of their visit. I enjoy working with patients and am humbled to be a source of comfort to someone in their most vulnerable moments. I eagerly strive toward ultimately expanding my impact through my work as a PA, and feel that my ability to persevere despite my life's challenges has prepared me for this most rewarding next step.

Appendix F:
Information About CASPA Waivers

The following excerpt is from the CASPA website, section titled Evaluations.[22]

The Family Education Rights and Privacy Act of 1974 (FERPA) gives you the right to access evaluations unless you choose to waive your right of inspection and review. Prior to requesting any evaluations, you are required to indicate whether you wish to waive your rights. CASPA will release your decision to waive or not waive access to your evaluators and designated programs. Your waiver decision serves the same purpose as a legal signature and is binding.

*Selecting **Yes** indicates to programs that your evaluator completed their evaluation with the understanding that you would not be able to view it. This means you will not be able to see the content of the evaluation. Programs may view this type of evaluation as a more accurate representation of an applicant's qualifications.*

*Selecting **No** indicates to programs that your evaluator completed their evaluation with the understanding that you may choose to view it in the future. Selecting this option does not allow you to view your evaluation via the application. If you do not waive your right to view the evaluation, you may ask your evaluator for a copy of the evaluation. Programs may view this type of evaluation as a less accurate representation of an applicant's qualifications.*

Once you make a selection, you can't change it, so consider the choices carefully.

---

[22] https://help.liaisonedu.com/CASPA_Applicant_Help_Center/ Filling_Out_ Your_CASPA_Application/3._CASPA_Supporting_Information /1_Evaluations

APPENDIX G: MY BIO FOR LORS

Samora Charles is the oldest of four children born to Haitian/Cuban immigrant parents. At a very young age, her parents instilled in her the values and importance of hard work and education. Her parents wanted their children to know that in order to be successful in life, one needed to take schooling very seriously.

Because of her parents' training, Samora developed an appetite for learning and enjoyed going to school. She was an above average student throughout her elementary and high school years. Her favorite subjects in school were always science and English. She particularly enjoyed biology and became fascinated with learning about the inner workings of the human body. She decided that she would major in biology in college, and focus on pursuing a career in medicine as a physician assistant. Her friends and family supported her and thought she would be a great clinician specifically because she was a very compassionate and altruistic person by nature.

During her freshman year of college, Samora had a disagreement with her family pertaining to religious beliefs and family structure. Unfortunately, this disagreement could not be resolved, and Samora was estranged from her family. Although she tried to move on with her life and ignore her feelings of rejection and abandonment, she suffered emotionally and her grades and health started to deteriorate. These unfortunate circumstances eventually led to her academic dismissal from Stonybrook University during her sophomore year of college.

Samora decided it would be best to refrain from re-enrolling in school until she had completely worked through her personal issues. During this time, Samora went to Uganda to visit a close friend who was involved in an educational enrichment program called Educate! for Ugandan children. Samora stayed there for a few months and worked for Educate! Most of the children enrolled in the program lived in villages that either had no schools or went to schools that were inadequate. These kids enjoyed coming to Educate! and it reminded Samora of how she used to be. She began to miss school and decided that it was time for her to go back and finish her education.

While in Africa, Samora got an up close and personal look at how disease and sickness prevailed in most of the poor communities in Uganda. Most people had no access to healthcare and lacked the resources that would allow them to treat and prevent disease. This bothered Samora and reaffirmed her desire to work in healthcare so that she can positively impact the health of others.

On May 27, 2013, Samora graduated with a 3.0 GPA and BS in Biology from CUNY City College of NY. She subsequently completed a post-baccalaureate at Medgar Evers College with a focus on upper division science classes, earning a cumulative GPA of 3.6. Currently she is enrolled in an MPH program at SUNY Downstate Medical Center. She feels that an MPH will help her become a more well-rounded PA as she will gain the knowledge and skills necessary to help others on a grander scale. In conclusion, Samora has persevered despite her life's challenges, and remains steadfast in her dream to become a physician assistant.

Appendix H: Standardized Testing Websites

GRE	https://www.ets.org/gre
PA-CAT	https://www.pa-cat.com/
CASPER	https://takealtus.com/casper/

APPENDIX I:
REJECTION LETTERS

Weill Cornell Graduate School
of Medical Sciences

Gary A. Koretzky, MD, PhD
Dean, Weill Cornell Graduate School
Senior Associate Dean for Research, Weill Cornell Medical College

Weill Cornell Medical College
1300 York Avenue, Box 65
New York, NY 10065

Telephone: 212-746-1361
E-mail: GradDean@med.cornell.edu

January 22, 2016

Samora Charles
1843 Prospect Place
Brooklyn, NY 11233

Dear Ms. Charles:

Thank you for your interest in the Master of Science in Health Sciences for Physician Assistants of the Weill Cornell Graduate School of Medical Sciences. I regret to inform you, that the Admissions Committee has not recommended the acceptance of your application for admission. I am sure you understand that our Program receives many more applicants than we can hope to place.

We wish you the best of luck in the future.

Sincerely,

Gary A. Koretzky, M.D., Ph.D.
Dean, Weill Cornell Graduate School

GAK:ab

cc: Katherine A. Hajjar, M.D., Program Chair
Gerard J. Marciano, Ed.D, PA-C, Program Director

Medical College Division — Sloan-Kettering Division

February 24, 2017

Samora Charles
650 Potomac Ave Apt 143
Alexandria, VA 22301

Dear Samora,

Thank you for your interest and application to the Physician Assistant program at Charles R. Drew University of Medicine and Science (CDU).

After careful consideration of your application, the program's admissions committee regrets to inform you that we are unable to offer you admission at this time. Admission to CDU programs is competitive, and meeting the minimum requirements for admission does not guarantee acceptance to a program.

Every application goes through extensive reviews, and the University regrets that we are unable to offer admission to all qualified applicants.

We thank you for your interest in the Physician Assistant program and wish you success with academic and career endeavors.

Sincerely,

Amin Maghsoodi
Director of Enrollment Management

CHARLES R. DREW UNIVERSITY OF MEDICINE AND SCIENCE
OFFICE OF ENROLLMENT MANAGEMENT
1731 EAST 120TH STREET, LOS ANGELES, CA 90059
PHONE: (323) 563-4839 FAX: (323) 563-4837

ARCADIA UNIVERSITY

August 5, 2015

Samora Charles
1843 Prospect Place
Brooklyn, NY 11233

Dear Samora,

The Admissions Committee of the Physician Assistant Program at Arcadia University has carefully reviewed your application for admission to our 2016 class. Due to a significant increase in application volume and the extraordinarily gifted pool of applicants we received, the selection process was extremely competitive. The Committee has reviewed your application and supporting credentials and determined that you will not be offered admission to the class. The decision regarding your application does not indicate that you would not succeed in Physician Assistant Studies; it only means that at this time your credentials are not competitive with the students offered admission. This decision pertains to our Glenside, PA and Christiana, DE campuses.

If you decide to re-apply you will need to complete a new CASPA application for the next academic year. If you desire additional information, please feel free to contact the Office of Enrollment Management.

Sincerely yours,

Diana Noller, MSPT, MMS, PA-C
Chair, Dept. of Medical Science and Community Health

TOLL-FREE: 1.877.ARCADIA (1.877.272.2342) • FAX: 215.572.4049 • E-MAIL: ADMISS@ARCADIA.EDU
450 S. EASTON ROAD, GLENSIDE, PA 19038-3295 • WWW.ARCADIA.EDU
A DISTINCTIVELY GLOBAL, INTEGRATIVE, PERSONAL LEARNING EXPERIENCE

ALBANY
MEDICAL
COLLEGE

Center for Physician Assistant Studies
47 New Scotland Avenue, MC-4
Albany, NY 12208

Offices: 16 New Scotland Avenue, Suite 264

Phone: (518) 262-5251 www.amc.edu/pa Fax: (518) 262-0484

September 11, 2014

Samora Charles
367 East 201st, Apt. C1
Bronx, NY 10456

Dear Samora,

Thank you for your interest in the Albany Medical College Center for Physician Assistant Studies. We are pleased that you want to become a Physician Assistant. Unfortunately, we are unable to offer you a position in our next entering class.

Admissions to PA Programs are highly competitive. If you wish to reapply for the next cycle you should consult with the admissions coordinator.

Best wishes with your career goals.

Sincerely,

Admissions Committee
Center for Physician Assistant Studies

Training the best physician assistants for over forty years

letterE9/11/14

Idaho State
UNIVERSITY

Division of Health Sciences
Office of Medical and Oral Health
Physician Assistant Studies
921 South 8th Avenue, Stop 8253 • Pocatello, Idaho 83209-8253

December 10, 2015

Samora Charles
1843 Prospect Place
Brooklyn, NY 11233

Dear Samora,

The program has received over 650 applications for the current admissions cycle. For the 72 available seats, the program will interview approximately 140 applicants. To streamline the process of reviewing applications to determine whether or not to call applicants for an interview, the program uses a file score to determine which applications to send on for review. The file score is calculated using the prerequisite GPA and the Verbal and Quantitative GRE percentile scores. The calculation is: the prerequisite GPA plus the applicant's Verbal GRE percentile score plus the applicant's Quantitative GRE percentile score.

For your application I have calculated a file score of 4.09 (a prerequisite GPA of 3.25 + GRE Verbal Percentile of 63% + GRE Quantitative Percentile of 21%). I regret to inform you that your file will not receive further consideration for this admissions cycle as the program will not be reviewing applications with this file score.

Although this must be disappointing to you, please understand that the number of qualified applicants greatly exceeds the available seats in this year's class. If you choose to reapply to the Program, you must complete a new CASPA application and pay the required fee. You will also need to resubmit your Graduate School application, submit any updated official transcripts and pay the application fee. The deadline for these applications for the class entering Fall 2017 is November 1, 2016.

Please be advised that if you do reapply, the Admissions Committee will be especially interested in what attempts you have made to increase the competitiveness of your application.

We wish you well in your future endeavors.

Sincerely,

Ann Smalley
Admissions Director

Phone: (208) 282-4776 • Fax: (208) 282-4969 • www.isu.edu/paprog

Accredited by the
Accreditation Review Commission on Education for the Physician Assistant, Inc.

MEDEX Northwest Physician Assistant Training Program

December 17, 2015

Samora Charles
1843 Prospect Place
Brooklyn, NY 11233

Dear Samora:

Thank you for applying to the MEDEX Northwest Physician Assistant Program at the University of Washington. We have completed our application review process for the 2015/2016 admissions cycle and we are sorry to tell you that you were not selected for an interview this year.

The MEDEX admissions process is highly competitive, and it can often require reapplication in a subsequent year in order to reach the interview phase. There are usually several areas that applicants can work on to strengthen the overall application. We encourage reapplicants to speak with and shadow practicing physician assistants, research state and national PA associations, and engage in self-evaluation of the application. It is also helpful to thoroughly review the information in this mailing, on the web site, and in any brochures you may receive.

Due to a significant increase in the volume of applications we received this year, we are not able to offer individualized feedback to each applicant. Therefore, as part of our effort to assist applicants in the process of reviewing their applications, a general feedback document is enclosed. A thoughtful self-evaluation and review of this tip sheet will provide areas to focus on for improving the application.

Watch the MEDEX website for new and updated information on the 2016-2017 application cycle. We encourage you to look specifically for the reapplicant information session(s) when dates are posted on the MEDEX website. These offer an opportunity to discuss ways to strengthen your application and also hear from current students who themselves were reapplicants before being admitted into the program.

If you are unable to attend the reapplicant session but are considering reapplying to MEDEX in the next admissions cycle (May 2016 – October 1st, 2016), please review the website for new and updated information. The admissions cycle for classes beginning in 2017 will open in May 2016, and the final application deadline will be October 1st, 2016.

Thank you for completing the MEDEX application process. We wish you much success in your academic and professional goals.

Sincerely,

MEDEX Northwest Admissions Committee
MEDEX Northwest, UWSOM
Department of Family Medicine
medex@uw.edu

MEDEX Northwest
Division of Physician Assistant Studies

MEDEX Seattle
[illegible]
Seattle, WA [illegible]

MEDEX Tacoma
[illegible]
Tacoma, WA [illegible]
253-[illegible]

MEDEX Spokane
[illegible]
Spokane, WA [illegible]

MEDEX Alaska / UAA
[illegible]
Anchorage, AK [illegible]

APPENDIX J:
ACCEPTANCE LETTER

HARDING
UNIVERSITY

PHYSICIAN ASSISTANT PROGRAM
Box 12231 · Searcy, AR 72149-5615
501-279-5642

Dear Samora,

Congratulations! The faculty and staff of the Harding University Physician Assistant Program are pleased to accept your application for enrollment as a student in our Class of 2019. You have worked hard to get to this point and we would be honored to have you join us in this remarkable journey.

We, as a faculty and staff of the Program continue to remain busy preparing for the exciting first day of class. August 14, 2017. Upon your acceptance of this offer, further information and details will be sent to you.

This offer will remain open for your acceptance until the specified date. To accept this position:

- ☐ Sign and return the acceptance contract, 2 weeks from receipt of the email offer, with a non-refundable $500.00 advance tuition deposit. This will be applied toward your tuition. Please give us a verbal confirmation or answer within 10 days.
- ☐ Read, sign and return the second page of the Technical Standards document that is also included in this package. The copy is for your records.
- ☐ Read and complete the privacy release form. Return this to us with your other forms and we will enter your H# and turn this into the business office.
- ☐ Return **ALL** of the documents to us in the enclosed envelope (the one stamp is enough postage).

Your actual enrollment into the program will be contingent upon the program receiving an acceptable clearance on the criminal background check. This background check will:

- Be with a vendor of the school's choosing
- Is a requirement to complete the acceptance process
- The information to complete this process will be supplied during the spring term
- The cost is the student's responsibility. We will keep the cost as economical as possible.

Once again, **Congratulations!** We look forward to hearing from you soon.

Very truly yours,

Michael Murphy, MD
Program Director

FAITH, LEARNING & LIVING

Appendices

Made in the USA
Monee, IL
05 December 2024

72621106R00095